AN INTRODUCTION TO
MICROBIOLOGY FOR NURSES

AN INTRODUCTION TO MICROBIOLOGY FOR NURSES

Edited by

N. A. SIMMONS, FRCPath

Consultant Clinical Microbiologist
Guy's Hospital, London

(Being the Enlarged and Revised Third Edition of
'Bacteriology for Nurses',
by Geoffrey Taylor, MD, DPath)

WILLIAM HEINEMANN MEDICAL BOOKS LTD
LONDON

First published 1968 entitled *Bacteriology for Nurses*
Second Edition 1972

Third Edition 1980

© N.A. Simmons, 1980

ISBN 0 433 30301 8

Photoset by D. P. Media Ltd., Hitchin, Herts.
Printed in Great Britain by The Whitefriars Press Ltd.,
London and Tonbridge

Contents

Acknowledgements

I would like to thank my wife for the considerable secretarial assistance which she has provided, and also Dr Louis B. Quesnel for very kindly providing the line drawings from which the figures have been prepared.

Department of Bacteriology
University of Manchester

G.T.
January 1964

Preface to the Third Edition

When Geoffrey Taylor first wrote this book his intention was to provide nurses and others in medicine with an outline of basic bacteriology. He kept the language simple and restricted those sections on the fundamentals of bacteriology, for example the physiology of bacteria, to the minimum necessary for the understanding of the later chapters of the book. He preferred to consider together bacteria causing diseases in each particular part of the human body rather than to present systematic bacteriology and describe organisms genus by genus. Thus the bacteria responsible for infections of the respiratory tract were considered together and there were chapters on infections of the gastro-intestinal tract and nervous system. Only the common and important infections were included and no attempt was made to provide a comprehensive guide to all of the infections of man.

In this revised edition I have adhered strictly to Geoffrey Taylor's formula and although there are some changes in all of the chapters, wherever possible I have retained the original text. I have replaced the chapter on the destruction of bacteria with one on Disinfection and Sterilisation and another on Antibacterial Therapy, and I have rewritten the chapter on Viruses Chlamydiae and Rickettsiae. However the keynote of the book remains its simplicity and I hope above all that it is easily understood by those who are approaching the subject of microbiology for the first time.

Guy's Hospital   N.A.S.
London   October 1979

Chapter One

A BRIEF HISTORY OF BACTERIOLOGY

The first clear description of bacteria was that of a Dutch draper named Leeuwenhoek in the 17th century. Using a very simple form of microscope he was able to see objects which he called 'animalcules' in rain water, and in the scrapings from between the teeth. He noted that some were actively moving, and described stick-like shapes and spirals. He did not associate his animalcules with disease. The animalcules have since been variously known as germs, microbes, bacteria, micro-organisms or simply 'organisms'.

The observations of Leeuwenhoek were soon confirmed, but because it was difficult at that time to conceive of so small a life-form, a bitter controversy ensued. The rival factions argued as to whether the animalcules were produced spontaneously under suitable conditions—the theory of spontaneous generation, or whether like other known living things they arose from others like them. The argument resulted in experiments which often gave conflicting results. Thus bacteria could be found in sealed containers of meat extract which had been heated. We would recognise today that the heating was insufficient to sterilise. The problem was solved by Spallanzani, an Italian priest, who showed that if meat extracts were thoroughly heated for a sufficient length of time and then sealed they would not contain bacteria however long they were kept. In addition he showed that such meat extracts would support the growth of bacteria if these were later admitted.

With the improvement of the microscope the study of bacteria continued and many differing shapes were described. It was not however until the mid-19th century that significant progress was made. Pasteur, a French chemist, was engaged in an investigation into the faulty fermentation of wine. He was able to show that it was a microscopic organism—a yeast, which caused the fermentation whereby sugar was converted into alcohol, and also that the presence of a rod-shaped micro-organism was spoiling the wine. Pasteur next investigated a silk worm disease which was seriously damaging the silk industry. Again he was successful. He was able to show that a living microscopic organism (subsequently shown to be a protozoan and not a bacterium) spread from worm to worm and caused the disease. This observation led to the germ theory of disease.

That living organisms, invisible to the naked eye, could cause disease was not easily accepted, and many ridiculed Pasteur. However, Lister who was Professor of Surgery in Glasgow, took up these new ideas. He believed that the bacteria present in the air might be responsible for the very high rate of post-operative sepsis. He introduced the spraying of carbolic acid (phenol) solutions over the operative area and by this means greatly reduced the incidence of infection. This was antiseptic surgery and it led eventually to modern aseptic surgery in which the aim is to exclude bacteria rather than admit them and then kill them.

The next important name in the history of bacteriology is that of Koch, a German doctor. His first important investigation was into the cause of anthrax, a primary disease of cattle and sheep which sometimes infects man. It had been found some time before that the blood of animals suffering from this disease contained rod-shaped bacteria, but it remained for Koch to prove beyond any doubt that they were the cause of the disease. This fact was confirmed a little later by Pasteur who also discovered a means of preventing the disease. He had previously discovered that under some conditions disease-causing bacteria could be made innocuous and unable to produce disease if given to a susceptible animal. These are known as attenuated strains of bacteria. This discovery he applied to the prevention of anthrax. By giving injections of cultures of attenuated anthrax bacteria to sheep he was able to prevent them developing the disease when later injected with a culture of bacteria which would kill unprotected sheep. This was the beginning of the prevention of infectious disease by means of vaccines.

Koch continued to make important bacteriological discoveries. He introduced the use of dyes to colour bacteria and so make them more easily seen under the microscope. He also produced the first satisfactory solid media for the growth of bacteria. Up to this time bacteria had been grown in solutions of various nutrients. Koch made these solutions solid by the addition of gelatine. This enabled cultures of a single strain of bacterium to be obtained much more readily. He was able to demonstrate in 1882 that tuberculosis was a bacterial disease. In doing so he propounded his now famous postulates: that a bacterium should always be found in association with its own particular disease, that it should be isolated in pure growth from that disease and that if then given to a suitable animal should reproduce the disease from which it was isolated. This clear thinking was of great value in checking claims that a particular bacterium caused a certain disease, ensuring that the causative nature of the bacterium had been proven to the full.

In subsequent years the causes of many infectious diseases were discovered; leprosy, gonorrhoea, typhoid, cholera and diphtheria were all found to be caused by bacteria within a short time of each other. A further important advance was the discovery in 1888 that the symptoms of diphtheria were not caused directly by the bacteria but by a substance produced by the bacteria. This substance, known as a toxin, diffused throughout the body from the site of bacterial infection and was able to produce tissue damage. Six years later it was found that antibody to the toxin—anti-toxin—could neutralise the effects of toxin and could be used in the treatment of diphtheria.

It was found several years later, in 1898, that some infectious diseases were not caused by bacteria but by much smaller, microscopically invisible bodies which would pass through very fine filters known to arrest the smallest bacteria. These became known as filterable viruses or simply as viruses. They have since been shown to cause a large variety of diseases.

Progress in bacteriology was extremely rapid in the latter part of the 19th century and the following years saw much of the knowledge confirmed and extended; the detailed structure and physiology of bacteria were investigated, the ways in which animals become immune to infectious diseases were studied, and later it became possible to cultivate and examine viruses.

Perhaps the most important advances in the last 45

years have been in the study of viruses, virology, and in the advent and development of treatment with substances which will kill bacteria in the tissues and so cure many infections, antibiotic and chemotherapy.

Strictly speaking an antibiotic is a substance produced by a micro-organism which in high dilution kills or inhibits the growth of other micro-organisms; chemotherapeutic agents are substances which have a similar effect, but which are synthesised or made in the laboratory. However, the distinction is not always easy to maintain since some substances which were originally produced by micro-organisms are now synthesised.

Perhaps the best known chemotherapeutic agents are the sulphonamides, the first of which, sulphanilamide, was found to be the active component of prontosil, a dye which was shown to have a curative effect by Domagk in Germany in 1935. The sulphonamides used today are safer.

The best known antibiotic, penicillin, was discovered by Fleming in 1929, but it was not until 1940 that Florey and Chain in Oxford demonstrated its unexampled potency and potential therapeutic applications. Penicillin is produced by the mould *Penicillium notatum* and since its discovery many thousands of moulds have been examined in the hope of finding other useful antibiotics, but relatively few have been found. The chance of finding a wholly new antibiotic is now low and most of the recent advances have been due to chemical modifications in the laboratory of existing antibiotics, resulting in substances which have properties different from the parent compounds.

Chapter Two

THE BIOLOGY OF
BACTERIA

Bacteria are very widely distributed in nature. They are to be found not only in relationship to man and the animals, but in soil, in water including the sea, and in the air. Only a very small proportion of bacteria can cause disease of animals or of man, others may cause disease in plants or live independently of living things. Many bacteria perform useful functions by altering the chemical structure of substances so that they may be more easily utilised by plants; without this service most of the vegetable kingdom and indirectly the animal kingdom, could not continue to live. In medicine we are concerned only with those bacteria which cause human disease; it is, however, important to realise that the vast majority of bacteria are harmless to us. The biology of bacteria is considered under three headings: their structure—anatomy; the way in which they obtain their energy and use food materials—physiology; and the growth and reproduction of bacteria.

THE ANATOMY OF BACTERIA

Bacteria are extremely small living organisms quite invisible to the naked eye. Very strong magnification, usually provided by a microscope, is required in order to see them. The unit of measurement used in the examination of bacteria is the micron (abbreviated as μ) which is 1/1000 part of a millimetre or approximately 1/25,000 inch. Bacteria vary in size from 0·5 μ in diameter up to 10–12 μ in length for the longer rod-shaped varieties. Bacteria may be examined microscopically in the living state in suspension in a fluid when some types will be found to be actively moving (motile) and others still (non-motile). When examined in this way bacteria appear as almost clear bodies and details of shape are not easily seen. It is therefore usual to use a dye or STAIN to colour them. Examined in this way bacteria are found to exist in a variety of shapes, the commonest being either spherical or rod-shaped. These are named a COCCUS and a BACILLUS respectively. Others are in the form of a sharply curved rod shaped rather like a comma and are termed VIBRIOS, or are elongated flexible organisms twisted spirally about the long axis and are known as SPIROCHAETES (Fig. 1).

As well as enabling the shape of bacteria to be seen more easily, stains assist in the division of bacteria into groups. The two most important differential stains are the GRAM stain and the ZIEHL-NEELSEN (Z–N) stain. In the Gram stain the smear of bacteria is first killed by heating and then stained with a dye such as methyl violet or crystal violet. The bacteria all become blue. They are next treated with dilute iodine which deposits the blue dye within the bacterial cell and converts them from blue to a dense opaque black. The stained film is now treated with either alcohol or acetone when, in some types of bacteria, the black deposit of stain is removed whilst in others it remains. Those retaining the stain are known as Gram-positive, whilst those losing it are Gram-negative. It is usual to counterstain the film with a weak red dye so that the decolorised Gram–negative bacteria are visible as red objects. The difference in staining is related to differences in the structure of the bacterial cell wall.

The Z-N stain differentiates those bacteria which, once stained with the red dye carbol fuchsin, will retain the colour even after treatment with strong acids

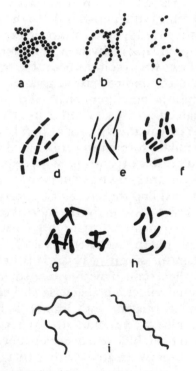

FIG. 1. The shape of bacterial cells.

(*a*) Staphylococcus, (*b*) Streptococcus, (*c*) Diplococcus (pneumococcus), (*d*) Bacillus, (*e*) Mycobacterium, (*f*) Escherichia (coliform), (*g*) Corynebacterium, (*h*) Vibrio, (*i*) Two types of Spirochaete.

and often also with alcohol. These are known as ACID-FAST (AFB) or ACID-ALCOHOL FAST bacteria (AAFB) and include the causative organisms of tuberculosis and leprosy. Most other disease-causing bacteria are non-acid fast.

The stains so far described colour the whole bacterial cell which appears as a uniform structure, but by other methods of examination greater detail may be demonstrated. The cell can be shown to consist of a rigid CELL WALL surrounding a central core of bacterial PROTOPLASM. By special techniques a structure may be demonstrated in the cytoplasm of rapidly growing bacterial cells which is believed to be similar to the nucleus of higher animal and plant cells. This has been confirmed by other techniques, including electron microscopy. It consists of a single circular chromosome which is made up of materials similar to those forming the nuclei of higher life forms, but differs from these in not being enclosed in a nuclear membrane. Like the nucleus of higher animals and plants the bacterial chromosome divides at cell division. The chromosome is made of deoxyribonucleic acid (DNA) and some bacteria contain smaller pieces of DNA in addition to the chromosome. These smaller PLASMIDS may confer on the bacteria amongst other things the ability to resist the destructive power of antibiotics. When this is the case the plasmids and the antibiotic resistance may be transferable, i.e. capable of being passed on to other bacteria.

Some types of bacteria are found to contain granules within the cytoplasm. These are thought to represent reserve food materials..

The cell wall of bacteria may be covered with a mucoid material which is known as the CAPSULE. It is probably secreted by the cell wall. The ability to produce capsules is often lost after prolonged growth in the laboratory, but is considerable in some strains freshly isolated from an infection. Figure 2 shows diagrammatically the structure of a typical bacillus.

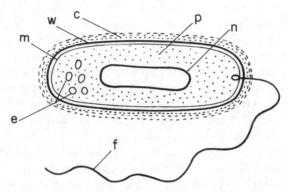

Fɪɢ. 2. Schematic drawing of a bacterial cell.

f—flagellum, c—capsule, w—cell wall, m—cytoplasmic membrane, p—protoplasm, n—chromosome, e—plasmids

Other important structures to be found in some bacteria are FLAGELLA (flagellum—singular). These are thread-like structures arising from the surface of the bacterial cell which by moving in an undulant manner propel the bacterium through a fluid medium. They may be arranged in various ways as shown in Fig. 3. Most bacteria not possessing flagella can only move by means of outside forces such as currents in the medium. The spirochaetes, however, are the exception to this rule, being motile by a corkscrew type of motion without the use of flagella. Flagella are not visible in the unstained state and special stains are required for their demonstration.

Some bacteria in the course of their life history produce another important bacterial structure. This is the SPORE. Spores are found as oval or spherical bodies within the substance of the bacterial cell. They have a thick, tough surrounding membrane which enables them to survive adverse conditions of heat or dryness which would kill the unaltered bacterial cell.

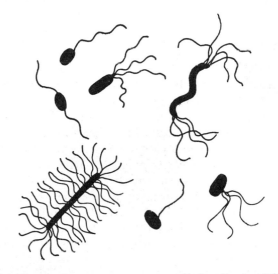

FIG. 3. The various arrangements of flagella in different species of bacteria.

When the adverse conditions have passed the spore GERMINATES and a bacterial population is re-established. Spores may be positioned in several ways within the cell (Fig.4), and may have a greater or lesser diameter than the bacterial cell from which they arose. Of the medically important genera only the rod-shaped species of bacteria produce spores.

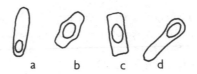

Fig. 4. Bacterial spores.

(*a*) Subterminal spore (Bacillus species), (*b*) Central spore (Clostridium species), (*c*) Central spore (Bacillus species), (*d*) Terminal spore (Clostridium species)

THE PHYSIOLOGY OF BACTERIA

In discussing the physiology of any living organism we must consider how it obtains the energy for its bodily activities and growth, how it obtains a supply of nutrients, what nutrients are necessary and how it removes waste products. Higher animals have complex organs for the absorption of food materials and for the removal of waste products; bacteria are able to carry out both processes by diffusion through the cell wall. The higher animals obtain their energy in a process of RESPIRATION by which complex chemical substances are reduced in complexity and energy is liberated. Oxygen is used up in this process and the complex chemical substance is said to be OXIDISED. The higher animals also use complex substances derived from other animals and plants to build up and repair their tissues. Bacteria obtain their energy in a similar way although in many bacteria the substances from which the energy is released may be simple in chemical structure, and oxygen is not always required. The entire food requirements of bacteria such as those living in soil or water may be only simple substances such as water and a mixture of simple salts. From these simple substances these bacteria obtain energy and build up their cell constituents. Many of the disease-causing bacteria require in addition amino-acids, proteins and sugars and other complex substances of animal or plant origin. This difference in food requirements is mainly due to the ability or lack of ability to make, or SYNTHESISE, more complex chemical substances themselves. Thus given a solution of simple salts some bacteria are able to synthesise their own bacterial protoplasm whilst others are dependent on having the building bricks of protoplasm already made for them.

Oxygen is not always necessary in the respiration of bacteria. Some bacteria are able to grow only in the complete absence of oxygen and are termed ANAEROBES, others will grow only with oxygen and are known as OBLIGATE AEROBES, the rest will grow under either AEROBIC or ANAEROBIC conditions and are called FACULTATIVE ANAEROBES.

Important sources of energy are the carbohydrates (sugars) which bacteria use by the processes of FERMENTATION and OXIDATION. These processes release energy and result in end products such as alcohols and simple organic acids together with carbon dioxide and hydrogen. Yeasts, which are fungi and not bacteria, ferment sugars in a similar way and are used in the commercial production of alcoholic beverages. It should be noted that fermentation is quite different from the way in which the higher animals use carbohydrates. Bacteria are often able to ferment a great variety of carbohydrates and tests of this ability are used extensively in their identification.

Proteins are also attacked by some bacteria. They obtain energy and also fragments of proteins which they may use to build up or repair their own protoplasm. In nature the bacterial breakdown of proteins is usually termed PUTREFACTION in the absence of oxygen and DECAY in its presence; both often occur together. These processes are essential in nature for the removal of dead organic matter.

In addition to the nutrients already mentioned some bacteria require the presence of traces of substances which can be considered in much the same way as vitamins in the higher animals. These are known as GROWTH FACTORS. Without the appropriate growth factor some types of bacteria will grow only poorly or not at all. The growth factors are substances which the bacterium cannot make for itself and which play an essential part in the physiology of the organism.

THE GROWTH AND CULTIVATION OF BACTERIA

Bacteria reproduce by simply splitting into two. Two new cells now exist where before there was only one. This type of reproduction is known as BINARY FISSION (Fig. 5). It is asexual and does not therefore involve the exchange of genetic material between two different bacteria. Genetic material may be passed from one organism to another during a process called CONJU-GATION when the two organisms are linked by a protoplasmic bridge. The recipient of the genetic material will acquire some of the properties of the donor bacterium and this may include resistance to one or more antibiotic.

The rate at which a bacterium multiplies depends on whether the prevailing conditions are favourable to the bacterium. Given ideal conditions a single bacterium may become two in as short a time as 20 minutes. At this rate about a quarter of a million cells will exist after six hours. The growth of bacteria does

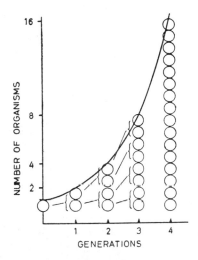

Fig. 5. The figure illustrates the rapid (logarithmic) increase in total cell population produced by binary fission.

not continue at this rate indefinitely. Food materials are used up and substances produced by the bacteria themselves are often damaging once a sufficiently high concentration is reached. These factors reduce the rate of multiplication until eventually more bacteria die than are produced and the total population falls.

The study of bacteria is most easily carried on in the laboratory by cultivating them under suitable conditions. Several factors must be taken into consideration. These are: (i) suitable food materials must be provided which will vary from bacterium to bacterium, (ii) appropriate atmospheric conditions which may be presence or absence of oxygen, and (iii) the temperature must be suitable.

MEDIA

The mixtures of food materials and chemicals on or in which bacteria grow in the laboratory are known as media. They provide the nutrients. They may be either solid or liquid, the former made into stiff jelly usually by the addition of a seaweed extract known as AGAR (or agar-agar). Nutrients are provided in many different forms; meat extracts, serum or whole blood are commonly used. In addition to providing the food for the organisms the acidity or alkalinity of the medium must be corrected and maintained correct by the addition of simple chemicals. The resulting media will be known as meat extract broth (nutrient broth), serum broth, etc., if liquid, or if made solid by the addition of agar, nutrient agar, serum agar and blood agar. Liquid media may be provided for use in either a screw-capped bottle or in a cotton-wool plugged tube. The cotton-wool plug acts as a filter and prevents the entry of bacteria from the air. Solid media are usually used as a flat sheet of medium in a round shallow

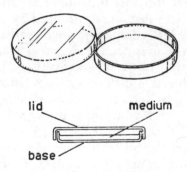

Fig. 6. The Petri dish.

The lower illustration is of a section of the dish to show the overlapping of the base by the lid.

covered dish known as a Petri dish. The top of the dish has a slightly greater diameter than the base and when applied prevents contamination of the medium by entry of bacteria from the air (Fig. 6).

Solid media are essential for the isolation of a pure strain of bacterium. The usual method is to inoculate one part of the dish of medium (usually called a 'plate'), and then to spread the inoculum over the remainder of the plate in the manner shown in Fig. 7.

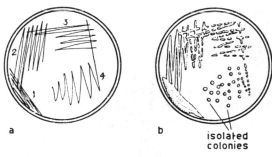

a   b   **isolated colonies**

FIG. 7. (*a*) Illustrates the method commonly used to inoculate a Petri dish of medium with a bacterial culture. The groups of strokes labelled 1–4 are performed in this order. The loop is sterilised by flaming between each series of strokes to avoid carrying over too many bacteria.

(*b*) Illustrates the appearances of the plate of medium after incubation. Note the isolated colonies from which a pure growth may be obtained on sub-culture.

In this way in some part of the plate bacteria will be present, separated from each other. After growth has occurred each bacterium will form a group; this when large enough to be visible is known as a BACTERIAL COLONY. Figure 8 shows the appearances of several types of bacterial colony. As the colony has developed from a single bacterium, a pure strain can be obtained

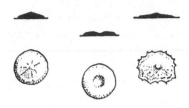

FIG. 8. The illustration shows the surface appearance and vertical section of three types of bacterial colony.

by taking a small sample from a single colony and re-culturing it. Liquid media are often used to investigate a bacterium once a pure culture has been obtained.

Many special media have been developed by bacteriologists for particular purposes. Some, known as *selective* media, are designed to stop the growth of some types of bacterium but to permit the growth of those which it is desired to isolate. Selective media are for instance used to isolate pathogenic bacteria from amongst the great mixture of bacteria present in faeces. *Indicator* media undergo some obvious change when particular bacteria are grown on or in them. These are used for identification purposes. Other specialised media contain food materials without which particularly fastidious bacteria will not grow.

ATMOSPHERIC CONDITIONS

As already mentioned (p. 13) the presence or absence of oxygen is of great importance in the growth of some species of bacteria. No special precautions are necessary when growing facultative anaerobic bacteria which will grow both with or without oxygen. In the growth of anaerobic bacteria oxygen must be removed and then excluded. The commonest method is to enclose the inoculated media in a sealed jar with a sachet which slowly releases hydrogen gas, which in the presence of a catalyst combines with the oxygen in the jar to form water. Some bacteria prefer to grow in an atmosphere in which there is a little oxygen and an increased amount of carbon dioxide. These are known as MICROAEROPHILIC bacteria.

TEMPERATURE

A strain of bacterium grows best at a temperature which is peculiar to that particular strain. This depends mainly on the temperature of the habitat in which it usually lives. Thus by and large it can be said that those bacteria causing disease in man grow best at body temperature, 37°C, whilst those living in soil and water will grow well at much lower temperatures. The temperature at which a strain grows best is known as its OPTIMUM temperature. In the laboratory this is provided by the use of incubators which can be set to maintain a suitable temperature.

At low temperatures below 0°C bacteria cease to divide but will survive in a dormant state for long periods. When the temperature is raised they again begin to multiply. Although some types of bacteria, notably those isolated from the water of hot springs, will grow at as high a temperature as 60°C, most bacteria are killed by exposure to this temperature for a sufficiently long time. Boiling will kill all but the sporing bacteria. Some bacterial spores are very resistant to heat and will survive 100°C, i.e. boiling water, for several hours. In order to kill spores quickly temperatures of 120°C are necessary.

Chapter Three

THE CLASSIFICATION OF
BACTERIA

Animals and plants are classified and given individual names so that in a discussion involving them the participants know exactly what is meant. Thus, in unscientific language, a lion or a buttercup mean more or less the same thing to everyone. Scientific classification goes further than this. It divides animals or plants into closely related groups and gives them all the same GENERIC NAME followed by a SPECIES NAME which is the animal or plant's own. Thus a lion is known as *Panthera leo*—*Panthera* is the generic name and implies that the lion is related to the other members of the genus, the tiger *Panthera tigris* and the leopard *Panthera pardus; leo* is the lion's own species name. Note that the name of the genus takes a capital letter whilst the species name does not. In addition to grouping into genera which contain only a small number of closely related living things, larger, less related groups may be formed. The contents of any group will have some structure or function in common. Thus the family to which the lion belongs is the *Felidae*, the cat family, including the domestic cat.

Bacteria belong to the group of life-forms which cannot with any certainty be called either animal or plant, although usually they are considered as very simple plants. Their classification is very difficult and although many systems of classification have been produced none is entirely satisfactory. The anatomy and detailed physiology are taken into account in their classification. An explanation of the details of bacterial classification is beyond the scope of this book, and all that is attempted is to introduce the names of some medically important bacteria. They are grouped according to shape and Gram-staining reaction and many of the less important ones are omitted.

GRAM-POSITIVE COCCI

Staphylococcus—Gram-positive cocci arranged in clusters rather like bunches of grapes; some types cause wound and other infections such as boils (see Fig. 1a).

Streptococcus—Gram-positive cocci arranged in chains; many strains live in close association with man; some cause infections such as tonsillitis and erysipelas (see Fig. 1b).

Pneumococcus (*Streptococcus pneumoniae*)—may live harmlessly in the upper respiratory tract of man; can cause lobar pneumonia or acute bronchitis (see Fig. 1c).

GRAM-NEGATIVE COCCI

Neisseria—Gram-negative cocci often arranged in pairs; some species found in the upper respiratory tract of man where they do no harm; two important disease-causing species—*N. gonorrhoeae* which causes the venereal disease gonorrhoea and *N. meningitidis* which causes a type of meningitis.

GRAM-POSITIVE BACILLI

Corynebacterium—Gram-positive bacilli which, when stained, often contain characteristic granules;

often arranged in groups rather like 'Chinese letters'; commonly found on the skin and other sites in man; some types, notably *C. diphtheriae,* produce a powerful toxin and cause diphtheria (see Fig. 1g).

Bacillus—large Gram-positive rods which grow aerobically and produce spores; widely distributed in nature in soil and water; only one member of the species causes disease of man (*B. anthracis* causing anthrax) (see Fig. 1d).

Clostridium—Gram-positive anaerobic spore-bearing rods; found especially in manured soils; some species cause gas gangrene and tetanus in man.

Mycobacterium—acid-fast bacilli difficult to stain by Gram stain but are Gram-positive if stained; some harmless species found in water and on grasses; two important human disease-causing species are *M. tuberculosis* and *M. leprae* causing tuberculosis and leprosy respectively (see Fig. 1e).

GRAM-NEGATIVE BACILLI

Pseudomonas—motile Gram-negative rods growing easily on ordinary media; produce green or yellow pigments.

Proteus—actively motile Gram-negative rods which often spread over the surface of solid media in the surface film of water; attack urea to produce ammonia.

Salmonella—Gram-negative motile rods characterised mainly by their fermentation of certain sugars; cause enteric fever (*Salm. typhi* and *Salm. paratyphi A*, *B* and *C*)and food poisoning (other species of *Salmonella*).

Shigella—Gram-negative non-motile rods; cause dysentery.

Escherichia and other allied organisms often called

collectively *coliforms*—Gram-negative rods normally present in the gastro-intestinal tract of man and animals; can cause wound and other infections (see Fig. 1f).

Haemophilus—delicate non-motile Gram-negative rods requiring special growth factors; can cause respiratory infections; the related organism *Bordetella pertussis* causes whooping cough.

Brucella—delicate slowly-growing Gram-negative rods; cause the chronic pyrexial illness brucellosis, also known as abortus or undulant fever and malta fever according to which species of *Brucella* is involved.

Bacteroides—Strictly anaerobic slender Gram-negative rods present in large numbers in the normal gastro-intestinal tract of man and animals; can cause serious wound infections particularly after surgical operations.

Campylobacter—Gram-negative microaerophilic rods. May cause food poisoning.

SPIROCHAETES

Treponema—delicate flexible spiral filaments. Difficult to stain by normal methods. The most important is Tr. pallidum, the cause of syphilis.

Leptospira—Tight spirals with hooked ends; the cause of a type of haemorrhagic jaundice (Weil's Disease).

Chapter Four

INFECTION

Only a minority of bacteria are able to cause human disease; the great majority live either independently of man or in amicable association with him. Bacteria which live in association with living things, dependent to some extent on them for nutrients and a suitable environment are known as PARASITES; those fending for themselves are known as SAPROPHYTES. Only a proportion of parasitic bacteria cause harm to the host; these are known as PATHOGENIC i.e. disease-causing bacteria. It should be noted that the division into pathogenic and non-pathogenic bacteria is not absolute: under some specially favourable conditions strains usually considered to be non-pathogenic may cause disease.

Man normally carries with him a large number of bacteria. These are known as the NORMAL FLORA of the body or COMMENSALS. Far from causing harm, disease may sometimes arise if they are deliberately removed. Their presence may make it difficult for a pathogenic organism to gain a foothold and in some cases they produce substances which are of use to man. Thus destruction of the normal flora of the mouth by treatment of the patient with broad spectrum antibiotics may enable fungi such as *Candida albicans* to grow almost unrestricted, producing oral thrush. Overgrowth of antibiotic resistant *Staphylococcus aureus* may take place in the intestine when broad spectrum antibiotics largely destroy the bacterial flora; staphylococcal enterocolitis may develop and may endanger life. Bacteria are to be found on the skin, in the mouth and respiratory tract, in the gastro-intestinal tract and in the vagina. The type of bacterial flora differs in these various situations. Thus the nose, mouth, pharynx, larynx and upper trachea contain Streptococci, non-pathogenic *Neisseria and Corynebacteria*, Staphylococci and Pneumococci; the bronchi and the lungs are normally sterile. The skin has mainly Staphylococci and *Corynebacteria*, but may harbour other organisms at times. The intestines contain very large numbers of bacteria. These include coliforms, *Bacteroides*, *Proteus*, *Pseudomonas*, *Bacillus*, *Clostridium* and *Streptococcus*. The vagina normally contains organisms which are able to live in the acid conditions prevailing there (Lactobacilli). The tissues and the body spaces which are remote from the outside are normally sterile. These include the nasal air sinuses, the middle ear cavity and the cavity of the uterus as well as the true interior of the body.

Infection is the result of the invasion of body tissues by micro-organisms. The body tissues may suffer severely or only slightly, depending on several factors. These are the local and general resistance of the body which are discussed in Chapter Five, the number or DOSE of bacteria gaining access to the body and the capacity the organisms have to multiply in the body and produce damage. The ability of bacteria to produce severe damage is known as VIRULENCE. Thus a large dose of a highly virulent organism in a person with low resistance will produce a very severe infection and probably death whereas a small dose of an organism of low virulence in a normal subject may produce only a mild, possibly unrecognised, SUBCLINICAL infection. There are many grades of infection between these two extremes.

BACTERIAL VIRULENCE varies considerably, not only from species to species but even in different strains of the same species. The factors which determine virulence in a strain of bacterium are not completely known but several are of importance. The possession of weapons of attack and the ability to resist the body defences both play important parts in determining the virulence of bacteria. Some bacteria having a capsule are less easily destroyed than non-capsulated strains. Perhaps the most important bacterial weapon of attack is the ability to produce substances which damage the tissues. These are known as TOXINS. Toxins may act either locally or be absorbed into the circulation and produce their damaging effects on tissues at a distance. The general effect of the production of large amounts of toxin by an infecting organism is known as TOXAEMIA. The local effects of toxin may be death or severe damage to the tissues around the area of infection and may seriously handicap the body defences. General effects include a raised temperature, general aches and pains, skin rashes and in some cases damage to 'target' organs. These are organs which are specially damaged by a particular toxin; thus the toxin of diphtheria damages the heart whilst the toxin of tetanus affects the central nervous system.

TRANSMISSION OF INFECTION

Infections may be derived from another person, animals or soil. The other person may be a patient with obvious disease or an apparently healthy person carrying the particular organism a CARRIER. Carriers are particularly important as sources of human disease, and may be difficult to detect.

After apparent recovery from an infection carriage may persist for days, weeks, months or years. For example, individuals have been known to excrete *Salmonella typhi* in faeces or urine for several decades after recovery from typhoid. Other carriers may be partially immune (see Chapter Five) and suffer from SUB-CLINICAL INFECTION. Nonetheless, they may pass on the infection to others, who may develop the full clinical picture of the disease. Carriers of *Staphylococcus aureus* are particularly important in hospital cross-infection. In patients with infectious diseases or in carriers, micro-organisms may be present either on the skin or in the urine, the faeces, the sputum or in discharges (e.g. nasal) produced as a result of the disease. Some diseases may be derived from animals. Salmonella food poisoning and brucellosis are examples of such infections. A few others such as tetanus and gas gangrene may be caused by microbes derived from the soil.

Whatever the source organisms must be transferred from it to a susceptible individual to cause disease. The methods of transfer may be subdivided thus:

1. by direct contact
2. by indirect contact
3. by air-borne transmission
4. by ingestion
5. by the agency of living creatures, e.g. insects.

The common modes of transfer of infection are illustrated in Fig. 9.

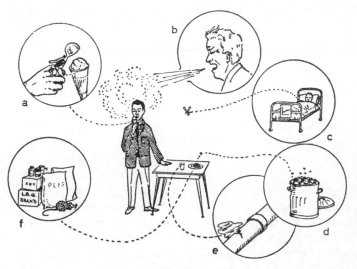

Fig. 9. The figure illustrates the different ways in which infectious disease may be spread. (*a*) spread due to food contamination by handling (*e.g.* food poisoning), (*b*) air-borne infection (*e.g.* upper respiratory tract infections), (*c*) insect-borne infection (*e.g.* malaria), (*d*) fly-borne infection (*e.g.* dysentery), (*e*) spread by contaminated water supply (*e.g.* enteric fever), (*f*) spread by animal contamination of food (*e.g.* food poisoning).

1. In the transmission of infection by direct contact pathogenic organisms are either placed on the skin or mucous membranes of the recipient or in some cases are directly implanted into the tissues as by a bite. Important examples of transmission by this means are the venereal diseases and in the case of direct implantation, rabies which is transmitted by the bite of an infected animal.

2. Spread of infection by indirect contact involves the contamination of some inanimate object by the sufferer; this then serves to pass the infection to

another individual. Examples of this method are the spread of infection by contaminated surgical instruments, glassware and crockery, blankets, clothing and many other objects.

3. Organisms are sprayed into the air from the upper respiratory tract during speaking, coughing and sneezing and others are shed from both normal and infected body surfaces. Bacteria are usually found attached to particles of textile, dried up secretion etc., and the smallest of the particles, droplet nuclei, can remain suspended in the air for long periods. In this form bacteria can be transported on air currents for considerable distances. They may be inhaled by a susceptible subject and induce disease or may fall on to a suitable site for growth, as on to a wound or a burn, and there cause infection. This type of transmission of infection is especially important in hospitals where patients may be shedding pathogenic organisms and many others will have wounds able to become infected. This type of spread is usually referred to as hospital cross-infection (see p. 35).

4. The transmission of infection by ingestion of pathogenic bacteria is the prime mode of spread of the infectious diseases of the gastro-intestinal tract. Food and drink may be the source or vehicle of transfer. Uncooked poultry or other meat is commonly contaminated with Salmonellae which may be carelessly transferred in the kitchen to cooked and otherwise safe foods thereby causing food poisoning. Other important diseases transmitted by ingestion include enteric fever and cholera.

5. In some diseases infection is transmitted by the agency of a living animal, perhaps the most important of which are the biting insects. The insects, by biting a

sufferer from the disease and then biting a susceptible person, carry pathogenic organisms over considerable distances. Human diseases carried by this means include plague, yellow fever and typhus. In addition the protozoal disease malaria is transmitted by certain mosquitos. Animals larger than insects can transmit infection. Rabies is a virus disease which infects dogs, cats, foxes and occasionally other animals. A bite from a rabid animal can cause disease in man.

HOSPITAL INFECTION

Infection is more readily spread from person to person in hospital than in the community outside for some patients are potentially a source of disease and others are particularly susceptible to infection since their natural defences are damaged.

Some patients are admitted to hospital because they are suffering from an infectious disease, such as diphtheria, which may be passed on to other patients or staff if adequate precautions are not taken. Patients who have had surgical operations will have wounds which are liable to infection with organisms which they or staff carry normally in the intestine or upper respiratory tract. For this reason particular care is taken to prevent the spread of infection in hospital.

THE PREVENTION OF INFECTION

The prevention or PROPHYLAXIS of infection is an important part of medicine as it is clearly better to prevent disease than to cure it once established. The methods used in the prevention of infection aim to eliminate the source and to interrupt the methods of spread discussed already under transmission of infection.

The most obvious way to prevent spread of infection by direct contact is to avoid such contact. Clearly this is usually impracticable as someone must inevitably nurse an ill patient. In serious infectious diseases, spread is limited by restricting contact to only those persons, nursing and medical, who are essential for the patient's recovery. Such isolation is usually carried out in a special isolation hospital.

Patients with less infectious disease may remain in a general hospital, but in a single room not in an open ward. They come into contact with as few people as possible who wear gloves when handling infectious material and gowns which are not allowed outside the immediate vicinity. In addition to prevent spread by indirect contact crockery, cutlery and instruments etc., which come into contact with the patient are restricted to the use of the one patient. Excreta and soiled dressings are treated with the greatest care to avoid possible contact with susceptible persons. Such isolation measures, previously termed 'barrier nursing', if carried out conscientiously are a valuable method of preventing the spread of infection, both by direct and indirect contact.

In any case of infection, even a mild one in which isolation is not considered necessary, it is essential that all contaminated material should either be destroyed or rendered safe by sterilisation or incineration. In addition all instruments, dressings, etc. used in the treatment of any patient should clearly be sterile and hence safe.

The prevention of infection by airborne spread is difficult since particles carrying pathogenic bacteria can travel for long distances. However, proper precautions may reduce the danger. Attempts can be made to diminish the amount of dust and to restrict its passage into the air, or the dust may be removed from the air as effiiciently as possible. Methods to restrict the amount of dust include the use of cotton and synthetic fibre materials for blankets. These shed far less fibrous dust than the more common woollen ones. In addition cleaning and bed making are not carried out before any treatment procedure which carries a risk of infection. Vacuum cleaners should be of the type in which some of the dust does not spray out of the machine after it has been sucked in. Furniture should be damp dusted. On no account should dry dusting or sweeping be allowed in hospitals.

Ventilation is the most important method of removing dust from the air of a room. It is however important that the dust is removed to the outside air and not transported to some other room. Ideally, positive pressure ventilation is used. In this method filtered air is pumped into the room and escapes from ventilators. As the air pressure is always slightly higher in the room than outside it, all air flow is outwards and infected dust is not allowed to enter. This method should be used in modern operating theatres. Ventilation by extractor fans or merely open windows carries with it the danger of replacing the air removed with air drawn from another more dangerous site. It is important to remember that the air leaving the room will be replaced from some other source which should not draw dust along with it. For example air should not be drawn into an operating theatre from a ward. The prevention of such occurrences is largely a matter of good hospital design.

Other measures that are of importance in reducing airborne spread of disease in hospitals are adequate bed spacing, a minimum of eight feet between bed centres being usually recommended, and the proper use of masks. These should be used in operating theatres, when open or extensive raw areas are being dressed or inspected, when carrying out minor surgical procedures and when attending premature infants. Small particles may pass from the mouth of the wearer through a mask but the larger particles will be trapped. Masks should never be temporarily lowered around the neck nor should the outer surface be handled since bacteria from the hands can be transferred to it and then be dispersed. The exclusion of known carriers of pathogenic organisms from contact with susceptible patients is desirable, but may be difficult to achieve since a symptomatic carriage of some organisms such as *Staphylococci* may be transient. However no one with a lesion such as a boil should remain in an operating room and before such a person returns to work the lesion should be fully healed. Hospital staff with chronic diseases of the skin such as psoriasis or eczema may be disseminators of *Staphylococci* and may be even more dangerous than staff with boils. Ruffling the hair disperses bacteria-carrying particles, and for this reason in operating theatres the hair should be completely covered with a cap made of an impervious fabric.

No one would knowingly eat or drink foods known to be contaminated with pathogenic bacteria and although without bacteriological examination it is impossible to detect such contamination, the risk of food poisoning can be diminished by good food hygiene practice. It is of great importance that food on sale to the public should be as safe as possible. In order to ensure safe food there are regulations governing its storage, sale, and quality.

Food may be contaminated directly from the animal which provided it, i.e. milk contaminated with tubercle bacilli from a tuberculous cow, or poultry contaminated with *Salmonella*. Control of animal health with the curing or more usually destruction of sick animals provides a means of reducing this type of contamination, but it cannot stop it completely as inevitably some animal carriers of infection are not detected, and in the other case the organisms which cause food poisoning in man are harmless to the animal. Thus *Salmonellas* may be found in up to a third of uncooked chickens from which it has proved virtually impossible to eliminate them. During processing or storage, food may become contaminated with bacteria from the air or from direct contact with man or animals such as mice, rats or insects. Animal and aerial contamination can be avoided by suitable containers and food handlers should be healthy and avoid touching food with the hands. Any bacteria present in food will be killed by efficient heating as in an oven, and many will be killed merely by boiling. The food at this stage is safe, but if left at room temperature may become contaminated and dangerous. To minimise this risk, cooked food, if it is to be stored, should be placed in a refrigerator. At refrigerator temperature most bacteria, though not killed, will not multiply. In kitchens, be they in the house or restaurant, care should be taken to avoid contaminating cooked with uncooked food. Separate utensils should be used for each category, or if the same ones are used they should be thoroughly washed in very hot water.

Uncontaminated water is often taken for granted in many countries, but water-borne epidemics have occurred in the past and still are to be found in some parts of the world. Water is normally treated by filtration in order to remove most of the bacteria. If the degree of contamination is high, chlorine may be added which chemically destroys bacteria. It is contamination after treatment which can cause trouble. A fractured water pipe in relation to a drain can pass bacteria directly into the drinking water. Control is achieved by repeatedly checking the bacteriological quality of water.

Transfer of infection by animals is usually controlled by attempting to remove the animals. In most cases this is not easy to accomplish. Thus although insecticides will reduce the population of insects, it is impossible to remove them all. If the disease in question is one which is confined to man, by denying the insects access to cases of disease the chain of infection will be broken. Both these approaches are usually employed together in preventing insect-borne disease. Rabies is an example of an animal-transmitted disease which has been controlled in Great Britain. The compulsory muzzling of dogs, now no longer enforced, and the quarantine laws, which prevent the entrance into the country of infected animals, completely eradicated rabies from Great Britain. Other countries have not been able to carry out these measures because of land frontiers and because of a wild animal reservoir of the disease. Unfortunately the risk of rabies returning is increasing because the disease in wild animals, particularly foxes, in continental Europe is coming closer to the northern coast of France, and thus closer to Great Britain.

OUTBREAKS OF HOSPITAL INFECTION

Outbreaks of infection due to one type of organism

which is readily transmitted and affects many patients can occur, particularly in surgical wards, in which many of the patients have wounds which may easily become infected if contaminated with pathogenic bacteria. The typical story of an outbreak of serious hospital cross-infection is that it is first noticed that the number of post-operative infections in a surgical ward is increasing. Bacteriological examination will show that many of the infections are caused by the same species of organism. In the case of some organisms, notably *Staphylococcus aureus*, which is a common organism involved in hospital cross-infection, it is possible to divide the species into types or strains. Typing is carried out by determining the susceptibility of the strain of staphylococcus to a range of bacterial viruses known as *bacteriophages*. These viruses are able to attack and destroy bacteria in much the same way as the viruses of human disease attack human cells. By using a large range of different bacteriophages (or simply phages) a PHAGE TYPE is defined which is characteristic of the strain of *Staphylococcus*. In the typical outbreak many of the organisms will be of the same type, and will often be found to be particularly virulent. At this stage of the outbreak of infection the problem is to attempt to discover the source of infection and the major method of spread. The organism may have been introduced into the ward by a patient who was already suffering from an infection, or was carrying the organism on admission, or by a member of the medical or nursing staff. The history of the outbreak may sometimes suggest which of these possibilities is the most likely. If a patient has introduced the organism it is sometimes found that the first cases of infection occur in patients whose beds are in the immediate vicinity of the offending patient. If a member of staff is the source of infection cases of infection may be traceable to a particular procedure carried out by that member of staff. It will often prove necessary in outbreaks of staphylococcal infection to examine nasal and possibly skin swabs from both patients and staff to discover carriers of the offending types of organism.

The mode of spread of infection may be by the air, or by direct or indirect contact. The history of the outbreak will again sometimes help in deciding which is the major route of transfer. Bacteriological examination of air samples may be useful in detecting air-borne spread, and a thorough critical examination of all techniques in use in the ward and operating theatre will sometimes reveal a careless practice which is spreading infection.

Once the source and mode of spread are known, attempts are made to remove the source by medical treatment or by isolation, and to prevent cross-infection by correcting techniques, improving ventilation, reducing or removing dust, etc., as already discussed under the heading 'The prevention of infection'. It may sometimes prove impossible to discover both the source and mode of spread of the infection in a particular outbreak. In this case the best method of control is to attack all possible modes of spread and so produce conditions in the ward in which further cross-infection is less likely to occur.

Chapter Five

BODY DEFENCES AGAINST INFECTION

The human body is by no means defenceless in the face of bacterial attack. Its defences can be arranged into two groups: non-specific, operating against a variety of micro-organisms, and specific directed against a single organism.

NORMAL NON-SPECIFIC DEFENCE MECHANISMS

1. The skin and mucous membranes
2. Phagocytosis and the inflammatory response

The intact skin provides a barrier through which most bacteria cannot pass. In this respect it provides a good defence against invasion. Most bacteria entering the body via the skin must do so through a breach in the surface or through skin which has been in some way damaged perhaps by prolonged pressure or friction. Some micro-organisms, for example the causative organism of syphilis, can probably pass into the body by the intact healthy skin. Sweat and sebaceous secretions by virtue of their acidity and possibly chemical substances have antibacterial properties which tend to eliminate pathogenic bacteria. The hydrochloric acid secreted in the stomach is also capable of destroying micro-organisms and will therefore prevent entry of many organisms into the intestinal tract. A substance known as lysozyme is present in many body fluids including tears, and respiratory and gastro–intestinal mucus which will kill some species of bacteria by dissolving away their cell walls. Bacteria are removed mechanically from the mucous membrane lining the respiratory tract. They are trapped in the sticky secretion on the surface, mucus, and then swept away by the action of cilia, minute hair–like bodies projecting from the cells lining the cavity. This defence system may be suppressed by cigarette smoke.

A most important general means of defence is the inflammatory response. This is a general reaction of body tissues to a noxious agent, be it bacterial, chemical or physical in nature. Following the entry into the tissues of an organism a series of changes take place. The small blood vessels increase in diameter and the rate of blood flow increases; the area becomes redder and warmer than its surroundings. The walls of the blood vessels allow plasma to escape into the tissue spaces and the white cells of the blood migrate into the tissue. This causes a swelling of the part. The white cells of the blood, together with certain tissue cells, move towards the bacteria and attempt to ingest them by a process known as PHAGOCYTOSIS (Fig. 10). In some instances phagocytosis may kill the bacterium, in others the white blood cell (phagocyte) may itself be killed. By surrounding the area of infection with plasma which often clots, and with phagocytes, the infection may be prevented from spreading. The flow

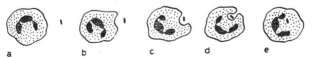

FIG. 10. Phagocytosis. The stages of ingestion of a bacillus by a poly-morphonuclear leucocyte are illustrated in *a–e*.

of fluid away from the area of inflammation is largely by means of the lymph vessels. Bacteria escaping from the area will usually enter the lymph and will be arrested at the nearest lymph node. Here a secondary inflammatory reaction may take place (lymphadenitis) but in many cases the infection will not become generalised. Thus the inflammatory response of the tissues tends to restrict the spread of infection within the body and in many cases to overcome it at the cost of a minor area of damage. If for some reason the inflammatory response is deficient, the infection will tend to become general and much more serious.

SPECIFIC DEFENCE MECHANISMS AND IMMUNITY

Someone who comes into close contact with a person suffering from an infectious disease may not contract it. For example only a small proportion of persons who come into contact with the highly infectious disease measles will contract the disease; the others will remain healthy. They are said to be IMMUNE to the disease. The term 'immune' is not necessarily as absolute as in the example given, and also includes the ability to defend against bacterial attack even though an organism succeeds in establishing itself in the body and produces symptoms and signs of disease. Immunity to infection can be conveniently divided into the resistance to infection which is inherent in everyone and that which is acquired by previous experience of the organisms or its products. Inherent immunity is known as NATIVE (or INNATE) IMMUNITY in contradistinction to ACQUIRED IMMUNITY.

NATIVE IMMUNITY

Many pathogenic organisms will only attack a limited

number of host species. Man does not suffer from many of the diseases which affect other animals and *vice versa*. Although not very well understood, the mechanism of resistance to infection with some animal pathogens is probably that human tissues do not provide appropriate conditions for growth. This prevents us from suffering, for example, from canine distemper. This type of native immunity is known as SPECIES IMMUNITY.

ACQUIRED IMMUNITY

It has been known for very many years that second attacks of some diseases are very uncommon. This is especially obvious in cases of the common childhood diseases. Two attacks of measles, mumps, whooping cough, chickenpox, etc., are most rare. The person is said to have acquired immunity by virtue of his previous infection. It has been found that following infection substances can be detected in the blood which are able to react with the infecting agent in question. The reaction is quite particular to the agent and no reaction occurs with others; it is said to be SPECIFIC in its activity. These active substances are known as ANTIBODIES. They are protein in nature and are produced in response to the entry of many substances foreign to the body. Not only the micro-organisms themselves but their products, including toxins, induce antibody formation. Substances which induce antibody formation are named ANTIGENS. Reactions between antigens and antibodies can be demonstrated in the laboratory by several methods. If a suspension of bacteria is mixed with the appropriate antibody, the bacteria will stick together in clumps—AGGLUTINATION. If the antigen is one in solution, the addition of the specific antibody will result in a combination of the two reactants, which under suitable conditions will precipitate out of solution—PRECIPITATION. In this instance if the soluble antigen is a toxin the resultant toxin-antibody combination will no longer cause the damage which characterised the toxin before the reaction took place. The antibody here is known as an ANTI-TOXIN. In some instances the mixing of a micro-organism with the appropriate antibody will render it unable to cause infection; the antibody is a NEUTRALISING ANTIBODY. In the immune animal antibodies can carry out other functions. Their presence can encourage the phagocytes to ingest bacteria and they also take part in the dissolving or LYSIS of organisms. Immunity to a disease may depend on antibodies which destroy or which aid in the destruction of micro-organisms or on antibodies which neutralise a toxic product of the bacterium. The former is known as ANTIBACTERIAL immunity and the latter as ANTITOXIC immunity. Which one or the other is the most important depends on whether the major damage caused by the disease is due to bacterial invasion or to the effect of toxins.

Acquired immunity can be conveniently divided into several types. The immunity may be ACTIVE, i.e. the antibodies are produced by the immune person, or it may be PASSIVE, in which the antibodies are produced elsewhere and are then given to the subject.

Active immunity depends on previous contact with the micro-organism or its products. Contact may be by virtue of a previous infection, overt or subclinical, or may be brought about artificially. Natural acquired immunity is of great importance in the infectious diseases of children. The child becomes immune to such diseases as measles, mumps and chickenpox after natural infection and such immunity normally lasts for the whole of life. Artificial immunity of an active type is used in medicine as a means of preventing disease. The body is presented with either the organism or its toxin in such a way that disease does not occur, but antibodies are produced and some degree of immunity is achieved. The bacterium or virus may be given as a suspension of dead organisms or it may be treated in such a way that although still alive it can no longer cause disease. Preparations such as these are known as KILLED VACCINES and ATTENUATED VACCINES respectively. It is possible to protect against some diseases by giving the patient a very mild subclinical infection which does no harm but confers a high degree of immunity against a subsequent natural infection. Vaccination for smallpox and live oral poliomyelitis vaccine are examples of this. If antitoxic immunity is considered to be the most suitable method of defence, the toxin is rendered non-toxic by various means and then given by injection. Toxins so treated are known as TOXOIDS and although they no longer produce damage on injection, they do induce the formation of antibody which will react with and neutralise the unaltered toxin. A single dose of an antigen induces the formation of only a small amount of antibody which in a short time disappears (primary response); further injections give rise to much more antibody and this continues to be produced, often for years (secondary response). Because of this a course, consisting of several immunising injections, is usually given. Preparations used to induce artificial active immunity are known as VACCINES. Artificial active immunity is available in the prevention of diphtheria, whooping cough, tetanus, smallpox, poliomyelitis, yellow

fever, cholera, enteric fever and others. The infectious
diseases in which artificial active immunity is commonly used and the types of vaccine available are
shown in Table 1.

Passive immunity may be acquired in two different
ways—naturally and artificially. In natural passive
immunity antibody is obtained by the young from the
mother either across the placenta or in breast milk.
The human placenta allows maternal antibody to pass
into the foetal circulation. The baby is then born having maternal antibodies against the diseases to which
the mother is immune. This provides the baby with
defence at a time when it is very vulnerable, i.e.
immediately after birth. The antibodies do not persist,
and after a few months will have disappeared. New
born cattle, and to a much less extent, humans, also
obtain antibody in the breast milk. This is absorbed
from the intestine and enters the circulation. In cattle
this is a most important contribution to survival, but
the amount of antibody obtained by the infant from
human breast milk is negligible.

In artificial passive immunity the antibody is
obtained from some individual or animal and is then
injected into the recipient. Antibodies to bacterial
toxins may be produced in animals, usually in horses.
After repeated injections of the toxoid, large volumes
of serum may be obtained from the horse which contains a high concentration of antibody. If this is
injected into man a temporary immunity will be produced. As a foreign protein the horse antibody will be
removed in a matter of weeks, but as a means of
combating the toxin of diphtheria, tetanus or gas gangrene it provides immediate protection whereas active
immunity would take weeks to induce. Horse anti-

TABLE 1

DISEASE	TYPE OF VACCINE	PREPARATIONS USED
Diphtheria	Detoxified toxin—toxoid	Diphtheria toxid—various preparations available, including ones precipitated with alum.
Tetanus		Tetanus toxoid.
Whooping cough (pertussis)	Killed bacteria	Suspension of killed *Bordetella pertussis*.
Enteric fever (typhoid and paratyphoid)		Mixture of killed suspension of *Salmonella typhi* and *paratyphi A and B* (TAB).
Cholera		Suspension of killed *Vibrio cholerae*.
Tuberculosis	Living attenuated bacteria (non-virulent)	Living suspension of the attenuated strain of *Mycobacterium tuberculosis*—Bacille Calmette-Guérin (BCG)
Poliomyelitis	Killed virus	Suspension of the three strains of poliovirus killed by formalin—Salk vaccine.
Poliomyelitis	Living attenuated (non-virulent) viruses	Mixture of living attenuated strains of the three types of polio-virus—Sabin vaccine.
Yellow fever		Suspension of a non-virulent strain of yellow fever virus (17D).
Measles		Suspension of attenuated measles virus.
Smallpox		Living virus of cowpox (vaccinia virus).
German measles (rubella)		Suspension of attenuated rubella virus.

body to tetanus toxin used to be commonly used in casualty departments to prevent tetanus in injured patients. However, persons who receive a large amount of a foreign protein may develop an illness, serum sickness, 8–15 days later with fever, a rash and swelling of joints. For this reason the use of horse antibody to tetanus has now been largely abandoned, but human antibody is used. If serum antibody is collected from a group in normal adults it will contain some antibody against most of the common infective diseases of childhood. The purified antibody preparation is known as 'gamma globulin'. This is used to produce temporary protection against the common infectious diseases in seriously ill and susceptible patients, and in protection against one type of infective hepatitis, hepatitis A (p. 130).

The acquired immunity described above is dependent upon the production of antibodies and is called 'ANTIBODY MEDIATED IMMUNITY'. Another type of immunity, CELL MEDIATED IMMUNITY, is dependent upon the reaction of certain cells, the T lymphocytes, to antigens. Cell mediated immunity is extremely important in maintaining resistance to many microbial infections in particular to tuberculosis and diseases caused by fungi.

HYPERSENSITIVITY

So far the interaction between invading organisms and antibodies has been considered; apart from serum sickness, the consequences to the host of an antigen-antibody reaction have been largely ignored. Most of the reactions between antigens and antibodies take place without causing any damage whatsoever to the host, but in some instances a state arises in which an abnormally great reaction occurs on presentation of the antigen. This is a state of hypersensitivity (sometimes referred to as ALLERGY). Hypersensitivity may manifest itself in several ways according to the type and to the way in which the antigen is presented. Two main types of reaction are found—the IMMEDIATE type where a reaction occurs within a matter of minutes, and a DELAYED type in which the reaction takes one or two days to reach its peak. The immediate type is antibody mediated, the delayed is cell mediated. Reactions in the skin to the injection of extracts of bacteria are used in the diagnosis of some diseases. The delayed skin reaction to tuberculin, a protein of the tubercle bacillus, is used in the diagnosis of tuberculosis. Not only bacterial antigens can give rise to hypersensitivity, indeed more important in medicine is hypersensitivity to pollens, foods, and other substances with which we frequently come into contact. The reaction which takes place between the antigen and antibody previously formed to it can give rise to such conditions as asthma, hay fever and urticaria. The antibody formed here is somewhat different from that so far discussed, and it tends to localise in tissue, such as the skin, the nasal mucosa and the lungs. When antigen is presented, the reaction occurs at the site of antibody attachment, release of active substances takes place, and these produce local damage to the tissues which is manifest in the symptoms of asthma, hay fever, etc. Tests for hypersensitivity to substances such as pollens and foods are carried out in the diagnosis of these conditions. By injecting small amounts of solution of the antigens into the skin, a weal will occur if the patient is hypersensitive. A full study of hypersensitivity is a subject in itself and is beyond the scope of this work.

DIAGNOSTIC SEROLOGY

As we have seen, the reaction between an antibody and its appropriate antigen is highly specific. This specificity is used in the diagnosis of infectious diseases of man by *serology* which is a study of antigen-antibody reactions. When an individual is infected with a particular micro-organism he will usually develop antibodies to the antigens present on the surface of the organism. Tests of the patient's serum may be carried out in the laboratory to detect these antibodies, and so we infer, if they are present, that the patient has indeed suffered from such an infection. Antibody studies are commonly used in the diagnosis of enteric fever, brucellosis, streptococcal infections and in many virus infections. The specificity of antibodies may also be used in the opposite sense. Specific antibodies, usually prepared by repeated injections of antigen into rabbits, may be used for the final identification of micro-organisms once they have been isolated in the bacteriology laboratory. Such specific antibodies will of course only react with the micro-organism which was used to induce the antibody in the rabbit. This technique gives a very precise means of identification which supplements the usual cultural studies carried out on micro-organisms.

Chapter Six

DISINFECTION AND
STERILISATION

The ability to kill bacteria is useful both in the curing of infections and in their prevention. If infection is to be avoided, objects such as syringes, needles, surgical instruments and substances which are to be injected, must not carry bacteria into the patient. Wound dressings and other materials which come into contact with vulnerable tissues must be safe and free from living organisms. To this end such objects are treated so as to STERILISE them. Sterilisation is defined as the freeing of an article of all micro-organisms. Disinfection is the destruction of pathogenic micro-organisms, but not necessarily spores. When bacteria must be killed we must consider not only the effect of the killing agent on the bacteria but also its effect on the object to be sterilised. Clearly, methods which may kill bacteria on a glass surface without damaging the glass may destroy a rubber or plastic object, or ruin a drug. From the patient's point of view, methods which may be be suitable for the sterilisation of surgical instruments would damage human tissues if used to kill the bacteria causing an infection. In the treatment of infections, substances known as antibiotics and antibacterial agents are used. These are considered under the heading antibacterial therapy. The methods used to sterilise inanimate objects are conveniently divided into chemical and physical types, and they are discussed under these headings.

CHEMICAL STERILISATION

Very many different substances have been used as chemical sterilising agents. This was especially so in the days before antibiotics, when considerable effort was directed to try to obtain substances which would destroy bacteria in infective processes without damaging the tissues. Chemical agents have been divided into disinfectants which kill bacteria and antiseptics which term is generally reserved for chemical disinfectants which can be safely applied to skin or mucous membrane to prevent bacterial growth. Disinfectants and antiseptics were often standardised by the Rideal–Walker or the Chick–Martin technique. These techniques compare in the laboratory the efficiency of a test agent with that of phenol, and the comparative activity is only tested against one bacterium, *Salmonella typhi*. These laboratory test methods are sufficiently unlike the uses to which chemical agents are applied in clinical practice to make the results virtually valueless. The In-Use Capacity test, which determines the degree to which a disinfectant can be diluted before becoming ineffective against several test organisms, is a more realistic means of assessing a disinfectant. In general, chemical methods of sterilisation are unreliable. The degree of contamination of the material to be sterilised and the presence of proteins such as serum, or pus, both tend to make the efficiency most variable. Chemical sterilisation should only be used in situations where physical methods are unsatisfactory, such as when physical methods would damage the object to be sterilised. The chemical agents discussed in this section include only those most commonly used at the present time.

IODINE and CHLORINE both actively kill bacteria, but they tend to lose activity rapidly in solution and in contact with organic substances, such as pus. Chlorine, usually as a hypochlorite which liberates chlorine in solution, is used to sterilise water where adequate filtration methods are not available. Iodine, as an alcoholic solution is widely used to sterilise skin. It is reasonably effective, reducing the bacterial population considerably, but rarely achieving complete sterility. Application of iodine to the skin of some persons may give rise to a severe reaction. 'Povidone-iodine' solutions are much less likely to cause reaction, are equally effective and more easily washed off. They are used for hand washing before operations.

ALCOHOL

There are several alcohols and isopropyl alcohol also known as isopropanol is the most effective. It may be used in an attempt to sterilise skin. It is most active when used as a 70% solution in water, but even at this concentration it is not very effective. It is best thought of as a skin cleaning agent rather than as a means of sterilisation.

COAL TAR PRODUCTS such as phenols and cresols are very efficient in killing bacteria. They are used in laboratories and for general disinfecting purposes. Many are caustic, producing burns if they come into contact with the skin. Derivatives of this group of compounds such as chlorxylenol (Dettol), which are non-irritant, are less effective disinfectants.

CHLORHEXIDINE ('Hibitane') and HEXACHLORA-PHENE are BISPHENOLS. Chlorhexidine has considerable antibacterial activity, and proves an excellent alternative to alcoholic iodine as a skin disinfectant. For this purpose it is used as a 0.5% alcoholic solution. It is also of value as an aqueous solution and has been used to disinfect non-boilable instruments, such as cystoscopes. Hexachloraphene is also used as skin disinfectant particularly in hand washing.

DETERGENTS of some types have antibacterial properties. Cetrimide (CTAB) is one such substance which has moderate activity. It is used in cleaning wounds, but cannot be relied on as a sterilising agent.

ETHYLENE OXIDE is a fairly new sterilising agent in medical practice. It is used as a gas in sealed containers, and providing the conditions under which sterilisation is carried out are carefully standardised, it is very efficient. It has been used in the sterilisation of pharmaceutical products and plastic disposable medical equipment, but not to any great extent in small scale hospital sterilisation.

FORMALDEHYDE was used as a vapour released from 'formalin tablets'. In this form, with or without gentle heating, it was used to sterilise objects which will not stand high temperatures such as catheters or cystoscopes, etc. Its efficiency is so variable that it should never be relied upon.

GLUTARALDEHYDE is a very effective liquid disinfecting agent. It may irritate the skin and eyes, but less so than formaldehyde. It may be used to disinfect heat sensitive instruments.

PHYSICAL STERILISATION

The physical methods of sterilisation include the use of heat, light, and of the ionising radiations X-rays and gamma rays. Physical methods of sterilisation are more easily standardised than the chemical methods and are much more reliable. Unless the object to be sterilised is likely to be damaged by physical methods they are to be preferred to control chemical treatment.

HEAT may be used either as dry or as moist heat, i.e. either with or without the presence of water or water vapour. Dry heat is the less efficient of the two types as bacteria are less easily killed if they are first dried than if they are hydrated throughout the sterilising process. Dry heat sterilisation may be achieved by heating an object to redness in a flame. This method can only be used if the object will stand this extreme treatment, but it is used to sterilise the platinum wires used in bacteriological culture methods. More useful is heating in a hot air oven. The usual type of oven is heated by electicity and can be set to give a desired temperature. It is essential that the set temperature is attained in all parts of the oven, and the best types have a circulator fan to ensure even heating throughout.

For sterilisation, high temperatures are required; 160°C for one hour is satisfactory, but sufficient time must be allowed for heat penetration and therefore it is simetimes extended to one and a half hours. Lower temperatures may leave the much more resistant bacterial spores still alive. At a temperature of 160°C many objects such as dressings, medicaments, plastic equipment, etc. are damaged and to sterilise such objects other methods must be used.

Moist heat sterilisation may be carried out in several ways. The simplest method is boiling. Boiling water at 100°C kills bacteria very quickly but does not kill all bacterial spores even if boiling is continued for several hours. It cannot therefore be said to be a reliable sterilising method. It is however commonly used because it requires only simple inexpensive apparatus and it is quick. It should be realised that boiling an object does not necessarily sterilise it and that the method should be used only if alternative sterilising methods are not available. The time usually recommended for boiling is 5–10 minutes. Another method employing relatively low temperatures is used to 'sterilise' objects such as non-boilable cystoscopes. This is sometimes known as 'pasteurisation'. This method uses water at only 70°C for 20 minutes. This treatment will kill the majority of bacterial cells, but of course will not kill spores. Using this method a calculated risk is taken: the risk that spores, if present, might cause infection in the urinary tract. Infections of the urinary tract with spore-bearing organisms are very uncommon and so the risk is generally considered to be justified.

Sterilisation by moist heat at temperatures greater than 100°C is carried out in an *autoclave*. This is a device in which objects may be heated in the presence of saturated steam at pressures higher than atmospheric. Temperatures higher than that of unpressurised steam, i.e. greater than 100°C, are thus obtained. The temperature at which water boils, i.e. is converted into steam, depends on the pressure of the surrounding atmosphere. Thus, although we are familiar with water boiling at 100°C the temperature of boiling water will be less than this at the top of a mountain where the atmospheric pressure is lower than at sea level, and conversely it will be higher than 100°C if the water is boiled at the bottom of a deep mine. We use this principle in the pressure cooker in which foodstuffs are very quickly cooked because a high pressure is built up inside the cooker with a consequent increase in the boiling point of water. The autoclave works on the same principle. It is important that the autoclave should contain steam without air because this both prevents the steam from entering porous objects such as dressings, and reduces its effectiveness as a killing agent. Nor must the temperature of the steam be raised above the boiling point of water. If the steam is superheated in this way the steam is far less effective and the autoclave behaves like a hot air oven. In order to kill micro–organisms the steam must actually reach them. If the dressings are packed very tightly, steam may not be able to reach the centre and the result will be unsterile dressings. If assembled glass syringes are treated by autoclaving, the steam will not penetrate into the thin space between the barrel and the plunger. The syringe will not be sterilised. If syringes and other similar pieces of equipment are to be sterilised by autoclaving, they must first be dismantled. Oil and grease on surfaces will prevent steam from penetrating. Equipment which requires greasing can only be sterilised satisfactorily by hot air treatment (160° for 60 minutes). Unfortunately hot air treatment may detemper steel and so damage surgical equipment.

Autoclave pressures have hitherto been measured in pounds per square inch (lb/sq in) above atmospheric pressure, but in future the gauges may give the pressures in different units. Unfortunately, all autoclave manufacturers may not then use the same units, but as, for the moment, they will all give the equivalent pressures in pounds per square inch I shall use those units here.

When working at full efficiency, without air, if the pressure above atmospheric in the autoclave is 15 lb per sq in the temperature will be 121°C, at 20 lb/sq in it is 127°C and at 30 lb/sq in it is 134°C. It is, however, important to have a means of measuring the temperature at the coolest part of the autoclave (the bottom), and not to rely entirely on the pressure recorder. The time required for sterilisation depends on the temperature achieved, and hence on the steam pressure. It also depends on the time it takes the contents to reach the desired temperature. Thus a large object takes longer to heat up than a smaller one, and hence should be given a greater time for sterilisation. An average time for sterilisation is 20 minutes at 127°C (20 lb/sq in above atmospheric pressure) with shorter times at higher temperatures and *vice versa*. The temperature and corresponding time selected depend mainly on the temperature which the object to be sterilised will stand without sustaining damage. Thus relatively robust objects such as dressings and most surgical instruments will tolerate high temperatures without sustaining damage; these may be sterilised at the higher temperatures—127°C (20 lb/sq in) for 20 minutes or 134°C (30 lb/sq in) for 10 minutes.

It is desirable to control the efficiency of any autoclave by testing its sterilising ability from time to time. One method is to insert into the middle of a typical load a 'spore strip'. This is a paper strip impregnated with particularly heat-resistant bacterial spores (*Bacillus stearothermophilus*). After autoclaving, the spore strip is cultured and if sterile indicates that the autoclave is working correctly. Unfortunately it takes several days of culture to be sure that the spores have been killed and the efficiency of the autoclave is not known during the interval. An alternative method is to place Browne's tubes in the middle of the load. These are glass tubes, the contents of which change colour if they have been exposed to a particular temperature for a certain time. Tubes are available for the common times and temperatures used in routine work. Browne's tubes have the advantage of simplicity but will not always detect autoclave failure because of steam containing air.

The most advanced types of autoclave carry out an automatic sterilising cycle. The autoclave is loaded and sealed, the air is then evacuated until the pressure is well below atmospheric pressure and steam is then admitted until the working pressure is reached. Because of the initial partial vacuum the steam penetrates into porous or hollow objects much better than in the simpler non-vacuum type autoclave. The autoclave is now held at the appropriate pressure for sufficient time and the steam is then removed to produce another partial vacuum. Dry, sterile air is now admitted which dries the contents of the autoclave. A continuous recording of the temperature and pressure changes is usually made on a paper chart. Examination of such charts will enable a faulty cycle to be detected and the material treated by that cycle to be re-sterilised. Prepacked dressings and sets of instruments are now generally processed in bulk in Central Sterile Supply Departments from which they are delivered to hospital wards and departments.

LIGHT, though bactericidal, is not a very useful sterilising agent. It has been found that direct sunlight will kill bacteria and that the portion of light responsible for this activity is the ultra-violet part of the spectrum. The disadvantages of ultra-violet sterilisation are its lack of penetration and the ease with which it is absorbed by such materials as glass. Ultra-violet light is sometimes used to sterilise the air of chambers in which materials are handled which must not be contaminated.

IONISING RADIATION such as X-rays or gamma-rays are active killers of bacteria, but a very large dose of radiation is necessary to ensure sterility of an irradiated object. They penetrate through objects fairly well and for instance will sterilise the contents of a sealed glass ampoule. Some substances are damaged by irradiation so this method of sterilisation is not universally applicable. Because of the dangers to the health of persons exposed to radiation and because the equipment for safe irradiation is both large and expensive this method of sterilisation is not suitable for routine hospital practice. It is however used by pharmaceutical companies and by the manufacturers of some types of medical equipment particularly for the sterilisation of disposable plastic hypodermic syringes and catheters.

FILTRATION is a physical method of sterilisation which may be used only with liquids. By passing a liquid through a very fine filter, bacteria are retained by the filter pad and the filtrate will be bacteriologically sterile. It should be noted that viruses are able to pass through the filters in common use. Filtration may be carried out in a Seitz filter which uses a thick pad of compressed asbestos to retain the bacteria, or in more modern filters which use thin porous sheets of a cellulose ester. Older methods, now rarely used, include the Berkefeld filter in which the liquid is passed through a column of the fine earth kieselguhr, and the Chamberland filter which filters through fine unglazed porcelain. Filtration methods of sterilisation are used when a liquid to be sterilised will not tolerate other methods.

DISPOSAL OF CONTAMINATED MATERIALS

Problems sometimes arise in hospital practice concerning safe means of disposing of contaminated materials. For this purpose the materials must be classified first into whether they are disposable, e.g. a pus-soaked dressing, or non-disposable, e.g. a contaminated surgical instrument or a hospital sheet contaminated with pus. Disposable materials are either combustible or non-combustible. Those which may be burnt, e.g. dressings, should be placed in a polythene bag, sealed, and then burnt in an incinerator. Those which cannot be burnt should be placed in a suitable container, autoclaved to render handling safe, and then be handed over to the local authority refuse disposal service. Disposable plastic syringes have become a large problem in many hospitals. Although they may be burnt with difficulty, the smell produced is offensive and the melting plastic tends to impare the efficiency of the incinerator. If they are to be burnt a suitable incinerator must be employed and the plastic burnt together with more combustible material.

Objects and materials which are required for further use are usually either metallic, e.g. instruments, or textiles, e.g. sheets, trays covers, etc. In dealing with contaminated re-usable objects, it is important to decide whether handling them is likely to constitute a hazard. A useful classification of contaminated objects divides them into:

(*a*) *Dirty*—no hazard to handlers, as for example a used bed sheet from the bed of a non-infectious patient.

(*b*) *Foul*—grossly dirty, as for example bed linen soiled with faeces from a non-infectious patient.

Though no hazard is involved in handling foul linen, most persons would find it offensive.

(c) *Infected*—contaminatedwith micro-organisms which may well cause infection in a handler. Objects, bed linen, instruments, etc., used in connection with patients suffering from infectious disease should be included in this group.

Dirty surgical instruments are normally washed before they are assembled and autoclaved for use on another patient. However, if they have been used on a patient with an infectious disease such as hepatitis and therefore are themselves infected they should also be autoclaved immediately after use to render them safe to handle and wash.

LAUNDRY

The washing process is a good hospital laundry should render infected linen safe. However, foul and infected linen should be bagged and labelled clearly and sent separately to the laundry. These precautions will be taken to prevent the laundry workers from handling it in an unsafe manner.

Chapter Seven

ANTIBACTERIAL THERAPY

The aim of antibacterial therapy is to treat a patient with a substance which will kill the bacteria causing an infection without at the same time damaging the patient's own tissues. Substances which may achieve this fall into two groups: those made by strictly chemical means—known usually as CHEMOTHERAPEUTIC AGENTS, and those which are made by living micro-organisms—the ANTIBIOTICS. For reasons discussed in Chapter One the distinction is somewhat artificial, but chemotherapeutic agents are usually much simpler substances than antibiotics. No chemotherapeutic agent or antibiotic is available which will be effective against all types of bacteria. The type or types of bacteria against which a material has activity is known as its ANTIBACTERIAL SPECTRUM. Even if an antibacterial agent is found to be effective against a number of strains of a particular species of organism it does not follow that it will be equally effective against all strains of that organism. It is the rule rather than the exception that some strains of a usually sensitive species will be found to be resistant. In addition it is possible for a sensitive strain to become resistant either spontaneously or after exposure to non-lethal amounts of an antibacterial agent. The change from the sensitive to the resistant state occurs spontaneously by TRANSFER or MUTATION. The mechanism of transferable resistance was described in Chapter Two. In order to understand the importance of mutational change to resistance it is useful to consider an infection in which a change to resistance to antibiotic X has taken place in one bacterium. If a sample of pus is cultured at this stage and tested for sensitivity to antibiotic X the bacteria will be reported as 'sensitive to 'X' because, of necessity, only a relatively small sample of the total population of bacteria is in fact tested. If the patient is now treated with antibiotic X the majority of the bacteria, being sensitive to X, will be killed. The resistant bacterium and its daughter cells will not be affected by X and will continue to grow. A sample taken at this stage will now show that the organisms isolated are resistant to X, and the infection will not have responded as well as was hoped. If the surviving bacteria from the patient treated with antibiotic X was passed on to some other individual and there initiated a new infection they will be resistant to antibiotic X from the start. The use of antibiotic Y in this patient may select a strain resistant to both X and Y, and in this way multiple resistant strains are produced. Such strains are common in hospital practice because antibiotics are used in large quantities and the opportunity for transfer of organisms from patient to patient is high. In order to minimise the development of resistant strains of bacteria, antibiotics are sometimes administered in pairs on the basis that the chances of simultaneous mutation to resistance to two antibiotics at once are very much less than the chances of mutation to resistance to one only. In addition, limitation of the use of antibiotics to only those cases who really require such treatment, and the use in these individuals of full dosage courses will also reduce the incidence of multiple resistant strains of bacteria. Because bacterial resistance to antibiotics is common, it is important that the sensitivity of an organism isolated from a patient is tested in the laboratory to decide the most suitable agent to use.

Laboratory testing of the sensitivity of bacteria to antibacterial agents may be carried out by several methods. The one most commonly used is the 'disc' method and this only is considered here. The organism to be tested is cultivated on a suitable solid medium on to which discs of blotting paper impregnated with antibacterial agent are applied. The agent diffuses outwards into the medium thus stopping the growth of sensitive bacteria. The end result is that around a disc containing an agent to which the organism is sensitive growth will not occur, whilst a resistant bacterium will grow up to the edge of the disc (Fig. 11). Although this is a somewhat crude method the results obtained provide a satisfactory guide to therapy.

Antibacterial agents can be roughly divided into two groups according to whether they are able to kill organisms or only to stop their multiplication. The former type is said to have BACTERICIDAL activity and the latter BACTERIOSTATIC activity. The body's own defence mechanisms are usually able to deal satisfactorily with the non-dividing bacteria resulting from treatment with a bacteriostatic agent. If it is known that the patient's own defences are deficient it is preferable to use a bactericidal agent.

Antibacterial agents act by upsetting some important part of the physiology of the micro-organism. It is not therefore surprising that they do on occasions result in upsetting the patient's physiology. This results in a TOXIC REACTION. Toxic reactions to antibacterial agents vary considerably in type and severity, the mildest being nausea and vomiting, diarrhoea, and skin rashes, and the most severe being damage to the blood-forming elements of the body, with perhaps death.

Antibacterial agents may be administered in several ways. Most commonly they are given by mouth and are then absorbed into the circulation from the intestine. In the case of some antibiotics absorption from the intestine is poor and they may then be given by injection either into a vein or into a muscle. In the treatment of some infections where a high concentration of antibiotic is required in the tissues as quickly as possible, administration by injection is often preferred. Antibiotics are sometimes applied directly to an infective process using either a powder or some form of ointment. This is known as topical application. In most situations this method of administration is not to be recommended as it is usually relatively inefficient and it tends to lead to the development of resistant strains of bacteria.

The following are brief notes on the more commonly used antibacterial drugs.

SULPHONAMIDES are a group of synthetic substances, i.e. are chemotherapeutic agents which act by competing with a substance necessary for bacterial growth. They are bacteriostatic and though usually given by mouth may be given by the intravenous route if speed and a high level of activity are indicated. Streptococci, pneumococci, *Neisseria* and coliforms may be sensitive although resistant strains are fairly common. Modern developments in the sulphonamides have

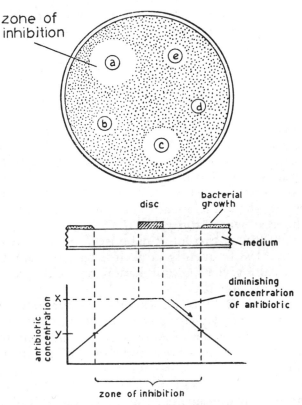

Fig. 11. The upper figure shows the appearance of the disc method for the determination of the antibiotic sensitivity of bacteria. The antibiotics are contained in the discs labelled *a—e*. Antibiotics contained in discs labelled *a* and *c* have produced large zones of inhibition of growth indicating bacterial sensitivity. Antibiotics *b* and *e* are surrounded by very small zones and antibiotic *d* is without a zone. The bacterium is resistant to antibiotics *b*, *d* and *e*. The lower figure illustrates the principles involved in the disc sensitivity method. Concentration *x* is the concentration of antibiotic incorporated into the disc; concentraton *y* is the minimum concentration which will inhibit growth.

resulted in substances which are only rarely toxic and which need not be taken as frequently as was necessary with the earlier compounds.

TRIMETHOPRIM is a synthetic substance which has an antibacterial spectrum that is similar to that of the sulphonamides. When given with a sulphonamide the drugs very often enhance each other's activity considerably. This mutual enhancement is known as SYNERGY. The mixture of the sulphonamide, sulphamethoxazole and trimethoprim in a single tablet or capsule is called Co-trimoxazole.

PARA-AMINO SALICYLIC ACID (PAS) is another synthetic chemotherapeutic agent which may be used in the treatment of tuberculosis. It is given orally and may produce gastro-intestinal upsets. For this reason it is used less frequently now. It is bacteriostatic and was usually given in combination with either streptomycin or isoniazid.

ISONIAZID (INH) is also a synthetic compound with activity against *Mycobacterium tuberculosis*. It is given by mouth and as with PAS is used in combination to reduce the incidence of resistant strains of the tubercle bacillus.

NALIDIXIC ACID and NITROFURANTOIN are both chemotherapeutic agents used in the treatment of urinary tract infections. Both are given by mouth and are concentrated in the urine. Both have antibacterial activity against many of the bacteria which commonly cause urinary tract infections.

PENICILLIN was the first satisfactory antibiotic. It is produced during the growth of a fungus and is hence an antibiotic. There are several types of penicillin produced either naturally by fungi or more recently by chemical alteration of a preformed molecule. The first type of penicillin to be used was BENZYL PENICILLIN, known also as penicillin G and as crystalline penicillin. This is given by intramuscular injection because it is destroyed by the hydrochloric acid of the stomach if given by mouth. It has activity against the Gram-positive cocci—the streptococci, pneumococci, and the staphylococci, but has little if any destructive action on Gram-negative organisms other than the *Neisseria*, which are very sensitive. Benzyl penicillin given by injection is rapidly absorbed from the muscle and very rapidly excreted in the urine by the kidneys, hence the time during which it is available to attack bacteria is very limited. It must be given every three or four hours. DEPÔT PREPARATIONS whereby the absorption from the muscular site of injection is much slower require to be given less often. PROCAINE PENICILLIN is a popular depôt preparation consisting of benzyl penicillin and the local anaesthetic procaine.

A variety of penicillin which may be given by mouth is PHENOXYMETHYL PENICILLIN or penicillin V. This has a similar range of antibacterial activity to benzyl penicillin but is not destroyed by gastric hydrochloric acid when taken by mouth. It is consequently used in medical practice where injections are inconvenient or undesirable.

Chemical alteration of the molecule of penicillin has yielded several useful penicillins. Only the more commonly used types will be considered. These are METHICILLIN, CLOXACILLIN, FLUCLOXACILLIN, AMPICILLIN, AMOXYCILLIN AND CARBENICILLIN. Many strains of *Staphylococcus* are resistant to benzyl penicillin. The resistance is brought about by the organism producing a substance—an enzyme—known as PENICILLINASE which is able to break down penicillin and render it inactive. Methicillin is not inactivated by staphylococcal penicillinase and is able to attack benzyl penicillin resistant strains. It must be given by injection because it is broken down by gastric hydrochloric acid if given by mouth, and should only be used if indicated by laboratory tests. Cloxacillin and Flucloxacillin have a similar range of activity to methicillin, again being resistant to staphylococcal penicillinase. They have the advantage of being active when given by mouth.

Ampicillin and amoxycillin have a much wider spectrum of activity than other penicillins. In addition to Gram-positive and negative cocci they will also attack many strains of Gram-negative bacilli, notably the coliform group and *Proteus* species. None of these penicillins is active against *Pseudomonas aeruginosa*, an organism which causes infections which are difficult to treat. CARBENICILLIN, the last semi-synthetic penicillin to be considered, if given in large doses is active against this organism.

THE CEPHALOSPORINS comprise a group of antibiotics which are related to each other in the same way that the penicillins are related to each other. They have the same central chemical structure, but chemical modifications have produced compounds with different properties. They are active against penicillinase producing staphylococci and Gram-negative bacilli except for *Pseudomonas* species. Some including CEPHALEXIN and CEPHRADINE can be given by mouth; others like cephaloridine and cephalothin must be given by injection.

THE AMINOGLYCOCIDES are a group of antibiotics which includes streptomycin, gentamicin, tobramycin and amikacin.

STREPTOMYCIN is an antibiotic which has activity against a wide range of organisms. Resistant strains of a 'normally' sensitive species are common, thus limiting its value. It is given by intramuscular injection, usually once or twice per day. Streptomycin has considerable activity against *Mycobacterium tuberculosis* and is often used in combination with either PAS or INH in the treatment of tuberculosis.

Toxic effects produced by streptomycin are not common if only short courses are used, but prolonged treatment results in damage to the eighth cranial nerve with resulting deafness and dizziness, which may be permanent. GENTAMICIN, TOBRAMYCIN and AMIKA-CIN are used principally for the treatment of infections caused by Gram-negative bacteria including *Pseudomonas* resistant to other antibiotics. They are not used in the treatment of tuberculosis. The toxic effects are similar to those produced by streptomycin.

CHLORAMPHENICOL is an antibiotic most usually given orally. It is a 'broad spectrum' antibiotic and is probably still the antibiotic of choice in the treatment of enteric fever. It occasionally produces very serious toxic effects, with the damage falling mainly on the bone marrow, with not infrequently death as the final result. Because of the known toxic effects of chloramphenicol many physicians only use the antibiotic where others are known to be valueless, and where without antibacterial therapy the patient is likely to be seriously ill or to die.

THE TETRACYCLINES form a group of closely related antibiotics all having virtually identical activity. The most important member of the group is TETRACYC-LINE itself. They are broad spectrum antibiotics taken most usually by mouth. Resistant strains of bacteria are not uncommon. Toxic effects are not usually serious—mild gastro-intestinal disturbances being the most common, but they are not usually given to children since they may stain the developing teeth yellow.

ERYTHROMYCIN is an oral antibiotic with a similar spectrum of activity to that of benzyl penicillin, i.e. it attacks the Gram-positive cocci, streptococci and staphylococci. It has been useful in the treatment of penicillin resistant infections but resistant strains of staphylococci are not uncommon and easily developed during treatment. It has no important toxic effects.

RIFAMPICIN is an oral antibiotic which has an antibacterial spectrum similar to penicillin. However, it is also active against *Mycobacterium tuberculosis* and it is generally reserved for the treatment of tuberculosis in combination with other drugs.

METRONIDAZOLE is an oral drug which has been used for many years in the treatment of vaginal infections with the protozoan parasite *Trichomonas vaginalis*. Recently it has been shown to be highly effective against the strictly anaerobic bacteria including *Bacteroides* and *Clostridium* species. It is not active against aerobic bacteria.

Chapter Eight

THE COLLECTION OF BACTERIOLOGICAL SPECIMENS

Bacteriological diagnosis is made either by identifying a disease-causing micro-organism in specimens obtained from the patient or by examining serum for specific antibody. Both methods of diagnosis are of course complementary. In either case it is of great importance that the specimens are collected correctly otherwise the results obtained will not be reliable.

General factors to be considered in the collection of specimens for culture are:—

(a) That the sample is from the actual disease process; for example, it is pointless to take a specimen of saliva if sputum is required and yet this is a very common mistake.

(b) The specimen must be examined in the laboratory within a fairly short time. This is important for two reasons. First, more delicate organisms may die rapidly at room temperature, and secondly some organisms may grow quite rapidly at room temperature thus 'swamping' slow growers and giving a false impression of the total number of bacteria in the specimen. Specimens which cannot be examined at once are usually best left in a refrigerator at 4°C.

(c) The specimen should not be contaminated accidentally. This could take place during the collection, be present in the specimen container or be added during transport to the laboratory.

Specimens of blood for examination for antibodies are usually required as clotted blood. Venous blood is collected and allowed to clot in a sterile container; the clot shrinks, expressing clear serum which is used for the tests. It is important that the specimen is removed from the patient using a *dry* sterile syringe and is later handled with care in order to minimise damage to the red cells with the release of haemoglobin (lysis). Lysed specimens can make certain types of antibody test difficult or impossible to perform.

Specimens should always be labelled carefully so that there is no possibility of confusion as to the source, type, and date of collection of the material.

The following notes give important points with respect to different types of bacteriological specimens.

PUS

Pus is best collected in a sterile bottle or tube if it is present in large quantities as is sometimes the case with an abscess. Care should be taken not to contaminate the outside of the container.

Smaller quantities of pus such as may be obtained from an ulcer or from an infected wound are best transported to the laboratory on a swab (Fig. 12). This consists of either a stick or a wire with a small amount of cotton-wool firmly wound on to one end. The whole swab is supplied inside a suitable container to avoid contamination. As much pus as possible should be soaked into the cotton-wool end of the swab; a rolling motion is often the best way to coat all surfaces of the swab. The swab should be returned to its container without touching the sides of the tube and the

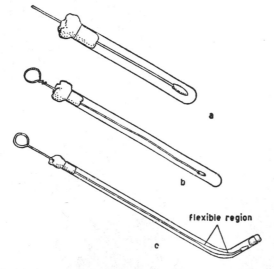

FIG. 12. (*a*) A general purpose swab, (*b*) a per-nasal swab, (*c*) a post-nasal swab (West's).

specimen labelled. Swabs may dry out quickly and bacteria, particularly *Bacteroides* species, will then die rapidly. To prevent this happening the swabs may be plunged into a sterile tube of semi solid agar, TRANSPORT MEDIUM. Most bacteria will survive for several hours in a suitable transport medium, but swabs should nevertheless be taken to the laboratory without delay.

Special types of swab are sometimes used. A PERNASAL swab is longer and more slender than the common swab and is passed through the nostrils backwards to the post-nasal space to obtain material from this site. It is sometimes used to obtain bacteriological specimens in whooping cough. Another method of approach to this site is the use of a POST-NASAL SWAB

(West's). This is illustrated in Fig. 13. The glass tube serves to prevent contamination of the swab as it passes through the mouth. Once in the post-nasal space the tip is pushed out and the curve on the glass tube directs it upwards. The tip should be retracted into the tube as it passes out through the mouth.

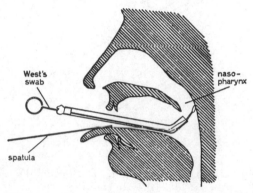

Fig. 13. Illustrates the method of taking a specimen using a post-nasal swab.

NOSE SWABS may be taken from the anterior nares usually to detect carriers of *Staphylococcus aureus* and THROAT SWABS usually from patients with sore throats or to detect carriers of *Streptococcus pyogenes*. Nose swabs and throat swabs are particularly likely to dry out and are best moistened with sterile water or saline before use.

URINE

Passed in the usual way urine is invariably contaminated by organisms present on the external genitalia. In order to obtain a specimen of urine suitable for bacteriological examination this contamination must be avoided or minimised. A specimen obtained by means of a urethral catheter is entirely suitable, but the catheterisation procedure suffers from the risk of introducing infection into the urinary tract. The most common safe method is to collect a MID-STREAM SPECIMEN OF URINE (MSU). This is obtained using either a STERILE funnel and a narrow-necked container or using a wide-mouthed container. The first part of the stream of urine is passed away, the next 50 ml. or so is collected, and the remainder of the urine is passed to waste. The first part of the urine washes away many of the organisms from the urethral orifice and so the MSU, although containing a few bacteria, is not heavily contaminated. Because of the slight contamination almost invariably present in the urine specimen it should be cultured without delay to prevent those organisms present from multiplying and so giving a false idea of the total microbial population. Mid-stream specimens taken from female patients are not as satisfactory as those from males, but if taken with care and if preceded by cleansing of the vulva do give adequate results.

FAECES

A sterile plastic container with a small plastic spoon attached to the lid is usually used. Faeces may be collected from a bedpan. Alternatively the patient may be instructed to float several sheets of toilet paper on the water of the toilet before opening his bowels. Sufficient faeces will be left on the surface when the patient has finished. The container should only be partially filled, and should be tightly capped to avoid spillage. Faeces may require to be examined for the presence of intestinal parasites; a similar type of specimen is used for this purpose except in certain instances. In the diagnosis of amoebic dysentery it is essential that the specimen reaches the laboratory within minutes of passing otherwise the typical movement of the amoeba will be difficult to find. After treatment of a tape worm infestation it is desirable to search the faeces for the tape worm head, so confirming the cure. In this case all the faeces which the patient passes must be examined.

BLOOD

Culture of the blood obtained from a vein is an important bacteriological examination carried out in infections of the heart valves, in septicaemia and in typhoid, etc. The blood must be obtained without contamination otherwise the result is valueless. The skin over the vein should be carefully cleaned with either alcohol or tincture of iodine, and an aseptic technique used to collect the blood. Immediately after collection the blood is injected carefully into bottles of culture medium which should reach the laboratory without delay.

SPUTUM

This is usually collected in a sterile wide-mouthed container. It is important that the specimen provided is sputum, i.e. is mucoid, mucopurulent or purulent, and is not saliva. It is best if the patient rinses out his mouth and if possible gargles before the specimen is collected. Some patients can't cough up their sputum easily and an experienced physiotherapist may then help in the collection of the specimen. Some of the organisms isolated from sputum are rather delicate and the specimen should be cultured without delay and not allowed to dry up.

CEREBRO–SPINAL FLUID (CSF)

This is required to be cultured in cases of meningitis. It is collected in a sterile container and should be examined as soon as possible. It is customary to place the first few drops which may be contaminated with blood in a separate bottle.

OTHER BODY FLUIDS such as those obtained from the pleural, peritoneal, pericardial and joint cavities are collected in sterile containers. The only points to note are that the containers should not be overfilled and that a small additional sample should be treated with citrate or some other anticoagulant to prevent the clotting, which sometimes occurs, from interfering with the microscopic examination of the cells present in the fluid.

SPECIMENS FOR VIRUS ISOLATION are collected in very much the same way as those for bacterial culture. Specimens which may be examined include faeces, throat swabs, blood, sputum, etc. It is advisable to consult the laboratory before taking any specimens since they may be best collected by laboratory staff. Throat swabs and other swabs are generally transported in a special medium which may be put into a very cold vacuum flask at the bedside. At any event all specimens should reach the laboratory speedily as many viruses die rapidly at room temperature.

Chapter Nine

THE PYOGENIC INFECTIONS

The responses of the body to invasion by a wide variety of bacteria are very similar. The body responds by an increased blood supply to the area and by an outpouring of serous fluid and white blood cells. This is the typical inflammatory response already briefly discussed in Chapter Five. The white cells which pass from the blood into the infected tissues attempt to ingest the bacteria (phagocytosis), many cells die and the resultant material consisting of both living and dead white cells (leucocytes or pus cells) and bacteria, together with damaged local tissues and blood proteins, constitutes PUS. Infections in which pus is produced are known as pyogenic, i.e. pus-producing infections. Pus may be present as a localised collection deep in the tissues—an ABSCESS, it may be produced on a surface, e.g. the mucosa of the pharynx, the mucosa of the bladder, the meninges, indeed any body surface, it is then known as a PURULENT EXUDATE. Alternatively infection may spread evenly through the tissues causing a diffuse inflammation CELLULITIS. The type of pus production will depend on the organism causing the infection, on the tissue in which the infective process is taking place, and also on the body resistance to the infection.

Although the pyogenic infections have very similar

appearances whatever the causative organism, different sites of the body have a tendency to be infected with particular species of bacteria. This is best illustrated by considering the more common bacteria associated with infection in different parts of the body.

WOUND INFECTIONS

A wound, whether surgical or accidental, has a tendency to become infected. The bacterial barrier provided by the skin has been breached and micro-organisms can pass directly into the tissues. This need not necessarily result in pus formation if the local and general body defences deal rapidly with the invaders. This means that potentially harmful bacteria may be cultured from a wound which is not purulent and which, even in the absence of treatment, never becomes purulent. However when the local defences are handicapped by the presence of severely damaged and possibly dead tissue and by blood clot, bacterial invasion is not resisted speedily and efficiently, and pus is produced.

A bacterium commonly isolated from infected wounds is *Staphylococcus aureus*. This is a coccus which is to be found in the noses and on the skin of a high proportion of normal people. They are healthy carriers of the organism. Unfortunately they may spread the organisms to sites in themselves and in other persons in which staphylococci multiply and produce an infection. Wounds, with their reduced resistance to bacterial invasion, provide very suitable sites for staphylococcal invasion. The organism may also spread from patient to patient during surgical dressing procedures in the ward. Staphylococci are also to be found in dust and may infect wounds by dust-borne spread.

Strains of *Staphylococcus aureus* which are resistant to many of the available antibiotics are not uncommon in hospitals. These are sometimes known as 'hospital staphylococci'.

Other organisms commonly found in infected wounds are those which are normal inhabitants of the faeces. These include the 'coliforms' (*Escherichia coli* and others), *Proteus* species, *Pseudomonas* and *Streptococcus faecalis*. These organisms are to be found on the skin of the buttocks, thighs, lower abdomen and sometimes elsewhere. It is not therefore surprising that wounds, particularly those of the lower abdomen, may become infected with these bacteria.

Two important types of wound infection are caused by bacteria of the genus *Clostridium*. These are large sporing rod-shaped bacteria which will not grow in the presence of oxygen, i.e. they are ANAEROBIC. They cause GAS GANGRENE and TETANUS. The Clostridia are to be found in soil and in dust; infection is always possible in a wound contaminated with such materials. In gas gangrene, infection with the particular species of *Clostridium* only usually takes place if there is extensive tissue damage, especially to muscle. The organisms produce much gas in their breakdown of the sugars in the tissues. The tissues become blown up with bubbles of gas which further damages them by interfering with the blood supply, in addition the bacteria also produces tissue-damaging toxins. The result of this infection is the widespread death of tissue—gangrene, with bubbles of gas.

Tetanus is caused by *Cl. tetani* which is able to produce one of the most potent bacterial toxins known. The actual area of infection is usually very small, indeed it may be insignificant. The wound is often a deep one but need not be large. The toxin produces severe damage to the nervous system, often resulting in death.

In both types of Clostridial wound infection actual pus formation is not marked, and may be completely absent in some cases of tetanus. They are included in this chapter because they are infections mainly of wounds, and on occasions the causative organisms are isolated from pus obtained from a wound also infected with pyogenic organisms. The use of antisera prepared in horses to protect against or to treat gas gangrene and tetanus has now been largely abandoned.

SKIN INFECTIONS

Two important types of pyogenic skin infection will be discussed which illustrate the different ways in which the skin and deeper tissues respond to infection with two types of bacterium. The organisms are *Staphylococcus aureus* and *Streptococcus pyogenes*. The two types of inflammation are the localised boil caused by *Staph. aureus* and the spreading infection ERYSIPELAS caused by *Strept. pyogenes*.

The boil is a common infection which almost always remains localised to a small area of skin. The infection starts in a hair follicle or a sweat gland duct; a pyogenic inflammatory reaction takes place and pus is produced. This distends the tissues locally but remains localised due to the toughness of the surrounding tissues and the very efficient inflammatory reaction. It is in fact a small abscess which usually bursts through to the surface and then heals. Sometimes there is some spread away from the original abscess which enlarges and then reaches the surface in several nearby points; this is a CARBUNCLE.

A completely different type of reaction occurs in erysipelas. Here there is no tendency for the infection to localise and to form an abscess. A typical pyogenic reaction occurs but obvious pus is rarely to be seen. Instead the infection spreads rapidly through the skin and subcutaneous tissues, and is seen as a diffuse spreading redness. The causative bacterium—*Strept. pyogenes*—has the ability to break down the tissue barriers which limit the staphylococcal infection just described and consequently spread continues until the infection is either treated or until the body defences gain the upper hand.

MENINGITIS

The coverings of the brain and spinal cord (MENINGES, see Fig. 15, p. 123) may become infected with a variety of micro-organisms when the result is meningitis. If the bacterium is in the pyogenic group it is known as PYOGENIC MENINGITIS. There is no basic difference in pus production in the meninges from that produced anywhere else, but because of its location the infection will sometimes produce very serious effects. Meningitis is an example of a pyogenic infection producing a purulent exudate; pus mainly is to be found on the surface of the meninges. Separating the brain and spinal cord from the meninges is a space containing a clear fluid known as CEREBRO-SPINAL FLUID or c.s.f. Into this fluid the leucocytes and bacteria escape, rendering it turbid. Examination of the c.s.f. as obtained by lumbar puncture is the best way to conform the diagnosis of meningitis. In pyogenic meningitis large numbers of leucocytes will be found whereas normal c.s.f. contains only very occasional cells. Also bacteria can often be seen in stained films. The important species of bacteria causing pyogenic meningitis are *Meningococcus* (*Neisseria meningitidis*), *Pneumococcus* (*Strept. pneumoniae*), *Haemophilus influenzae*, and in neonates coliform organisms and *Proteus* species. As these organisms have quite different appearances in stained films it may be possible to obtain a reasonably accurate preliminary identification within a very short time. Culture is necessary to confirm the diagnosis and to carry out sensitivity testing. The *Meningococcus* is killed by quite short exposure to room temperature and c.s.f. should therefore be cultured soon after collection in any suspected case of pyogenic meningitis.

URINARY TRACT INFECTIONS

The urinary tract comprises the two kidneys, the ureters, the bladder and the urethra. Commonly the two important sites of bacterial infection are the pelvis of the kidney and the bladder. These infections are known as PYELITIS (or pyelonephritis as the kidney itself is usually infected as well as the renal pelvis) and CYSTITIS respectively. Sometimes an ascending infection occurs which starts as a cystitis and moves up the renal tract to involve the kidney, in other cases the infection remains localised in one site or the other.

The bacteria commonly causing urinary tract infections are *Escherichia coli* and other related organisms—the 'coliforms', *Proteus* and *Streptococcus faecalis*. These are the bacteria commonly found in faeces, and already seen to be the cause of many wound infections, especially of surgical wounds of the abdomen. It is very unusual for the normal urinary tract to become infected spontaneously, but if other diseases such as tumours, congenital malformations, injuries, etc. are present infection often occurs as a complication. The infection may be introduced by surgical procedures such as catheterisation, or may occur without intervention, either by upward passage of bacteria from the outside, or spread to the urinary tract from the intestine by the blood or lymph vessels. One type of urinary tract infection worthy of note is PYELITIS OF PREGNANCY. In pregnancy the urinary tract cannot be considered normal; the obstruction to urine flow provided by the enlarged uterus, and the stretching of pelvic structures both increase the susceptibility to infection. The commonest offending organism in this type of urinary infection is *Esch. coli*.

Bacteriological confirmation of the diagnosis of acute urinary tract infections is relatively straightforward. Microscopic examination of a mid-stream specimen of urine will usually show the presence of many leucocytes, and culture will yield a heavy growth of the causative organism. Urinary tract infections may often recur in spite of efficient treatment and may ultimately become chronic. Diagnosis is then not quite so easy, as leucocytes may be scanty and only be present in the urine intermittently. Cylindrical masses of cells known as CASTS may be found in chronic urinary infections. Chronic urinary tract infections almost invariably involve the kidneys, and may eventually result in failure of kidney function.

PERITONITIS AND PLEURISY

In infection of the peritoneum and the pleura, both serous membranes, the inflammation takes the form of a purulent exudate. In more severe infections free pus is formed. This is known as an EMPYEMA in the case of pus in the pleural cavity. Peritonitis is usually caused by organisms derived from the gastro–intestinal tract. They reach the peritoneum often by rupture of the intestine as by perforation of a gastric ulcer, of an inflamed appendix, or by wounds, either surgical or otherwise. The organisms involved include those already mentioned under urinary infections. In addition anaerobic organisms will sometimes be isolated from peritoneal pus. These include the anaerobic Streptococci and bacilli of the genus *Bacteroides*. The organisms causing infection of the pleura reach this site by way of the lungs, secondary to pulmonary infection, i.e. pneumonia. The common organisms isolated include *Pneumococcus* (*Strep. pneumoniae*), *Staphylococcus aureus* and *Klebsiella pneumoniae*. Serious infection of the pleural cavity is no longer very common due to the treatment of pneumonia with antibiotics.

Infections of both the pleura and the peritoneum are commonly followed by healing with the formation of bands or sheets of fibrous tissue which join adjacent portions of the membranes together. These are known as adhesions. In the peritoneal cavity they may cause intestinal obstruction by being stretched tightly across a loop of intestine.

MISCELLANEOUS PYOGENIC INFECTIONS

GONORRHOEA is an acute pyogenic infection involving mainly the urethra in the male, and in the female also the cervix of the uterus. It is caused by the coccus *Neisseria gonorrhoeae*, the 'gonococcus'. It is a venereal disease, i.e. infection is spread from a sufferer from the disease to others by means of sexual contact. In the female there may be a vaginal discharge and pain or irritation on passing urine. The symptoms are more definite in the male in whom a purulent discharge occurs from the urethra. The Neisseria may be seen as pink oval cocci within pus cells when stained by the Gram technique. The infection usually responds well to treatment with penicillin, but if left untreated becomes chronic and may produce more serious damage to both male and female reproductive systems. Unfortunately strains of *N. gonorrhoeae* which produce penicillinase and are therefore resistant to penicillin have recently been described but at the moment they are relatively rare.

ARTHRITIS

Inflammation of a joint may be infective or non-infective, the latter type being by far the most common. Types of non-infective arthritis include osteo-arthritis, rheumatoid arthritis and the arthritis of rheumatic fever. Purulent arthritis, which is quite rare, may occur as a result of accidental or surgical wounds of a joint when the bacteria isolated are those already discussed in the section on wound infection. Bacteria may reach a joint by way of the blood stream when the arthritis produced will appear as a complication of another bacterial disease or as a sudden unexpected happening. In pyogenic arthritis there is an outpouring of fluid into the joint space which will contain many pus cells. Quite commonly there is considerable destruction of the structure of the joint, particularly of the joint cartilages. Bacteria which may cause pyogenic arthritis include the gonococcus, *Staphylococcus aureus*, and *Streptococcus pyogenes*.

    OTITIS is the name given to infectons of the ear. The

ear flap or pinna directs sound waves down the ear passage to the middle ear, a narrow cavity separated from the ear passage by the tympanic membrane (ear drum). Vibrations are transmitted across the middle ear by a set of small bones to the sensory mechanism of the inner ear. The middle ear cavity is connected directly to the back of the throat by the Eustachian tube. Infection of the middle ear is called OTITIS MEDIA. Acute otitis media usually follows a cold, influenza, sore throat or childhood illness such as measles. In children the development of the disease is favoured by the wide straight Eustachian tube. Organisms which may cause this infection are *Streptococcus pyogenes*, *Pneumococcus*, *Staphylococcus aureus*, and particularly in children *Haemophilus influenzae*.

Chapter Ten

CHRONIC BACTERIAL
INFECTIONS

The inflammation resulting from bacterial infection may be either ACUTE or CHRONIC. A major difference between the two types is the pace of the inflammatory response. We have seen in Chapter Nine that the pyogenic response occurs speedily; the disease process rapidly reaches a peak, and usually the patient recovers either with or without treatment or sometimes dies. The essence of acute inflammation is its speed. In chronic bacterial inflammation events occur much more slowly, the disease may continue at a low level of activity, slowly destroying surrounding tissues for months and years. An intermediate type known as SUBACUTE inflammation is also sometimes described, but there is considerable difficulty in deciding where its boundaries lie; it is perhaps best considered as prolonged acute inflammation.

By no means all chronic inflammation is caused by bacteria. Inflammation of a chronic type occurs as a result of repeated frequent damage to a part of the body, as for example a joint, also it may result from chemical damage to tissues. It is found in many well-recognised diseases, the cause of which is still unknown, but in which there is considerable evidence available to suggest that bacteria are not the cause.

The chronic inflammatory diseases selected for consideration here are syphilis and tuberculosis. There are certain similarities in these diseases; they result in the formaton of a CHRONIC GRANULOMA at some stage of their natural history. A chronic granuloma is an inflammatory process in which there is destruction of the host tissues with replacement by inflammatory cells and fibrous tissue. The inflammatory cell characteristic of the chronic granuloma is not the pus cell of acute inflammation but the large scavenging cell—the MACROPHAGE. In addition the LYMPHOCYTE, a cell found in lymph nodes, the spleen and in normal blood, is also seen in the chronic granuloma.

TUBERCULOSIS

The micro–organism causing tuberculosis is *Mycobacterium tuberculosis*. It is a rod–shaped, often slightly curved, organism and it may have a beaded appearance when stained. Gram's method fails to stain *M. tuberculosis*, and the ZIEHL-NEELSEN method is used (p. 8). The organism will grow on specialised artificial media, but is much slower to produce a visible colony than most bacteria already considered, about four weeks being required. Two main strains of *M. tuberculosis* can be distinguished—the human and bovine strains. The latter is frequently called *Mycobacterium bovis*. Both can cause human disease. The human strain of tuberculosis is spread from man to man most often by means of infected sputum—i.e. mainly by airborne spread. The bovine strain reaches man in milk derived from a tuberculous cow. The latter type has now been successfully controlled in many countries by the pasteurisation of milk and the testing of cattle for tuberculosis (tuberculin tested—T.T. herds). The two strains of *M. tuberculosis* tend to cause tuberculosis of different sites in the body mainly because of the difference in the route of infection. Human strain tuberculosis is most often of the lungs, whereas bovine tuberculosis usually involves the intestine and the lymph nodes of the neck.

In a population in which tuberculosis is common most persons contract the disease in childhood, so that by adolescence almost every person will show evidence of past or of active infection. In the vast majority of persons the infection is rapidly overcome and a measure of resistance to the disease develops. In such a primary infection a small area of inflammation occurs, most commonly in the lung, and the local lymph nodes and lymph vessels also share in the inflammation. This is known as a PRIMARY COMPLEX. The characteristic cells of chronic inflammation are found arranged in small roughly spherical groups known as TUBERCLES (Fig. 14). Healing takes place with only minimal destruction of tissue and all that remains is a tiny scar which may later become calcified. Because of the primary infection the person develops an increased sensitivity to an extract of the tubercle bacillus (TUBERCULIN). If this material is injected into the skin an area of temporary inflammation occurs, whereas it produces no reaction at all in a person who has never been infected with tuberculosis. This test is known as the MANTOUX test and is used to determine whether or not a person has had tuberculosis in the past. There are other variations of the test; one being the HEAF test in which a 'gun' is used to prick the tuberculin into the skin and another the 'TINE' test, in which the tuberculin is inoculated with a disposable spiked cone.

Occasionally the primary complex does not heal and spread may take place. The reason for the spread

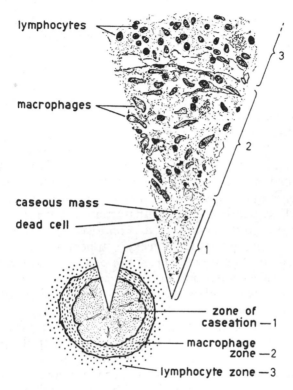

Fig. 14. Illustrates the microscopic appearances of a tubercle. Note the concentric arrangement of the caseation, macrophages (epithelioid cells) and lymphocytes.

may be that the sufferer has a very low resistance to infection, or that the tubercle bacillus was a specially virulent strain, or that the dose of bacteria received was large. Spread may take place locally with more destruction of neighbouring tissue, or the bacteria may enter the blood stream with the result that tuberculosis of many parts of the body occurs. Bloodstream spread tuberculosis is known as MILIARY TUBERCULOSIS. Many organs will develop tiny MILI-ARY TUBERCLES, the patient will become very ill and may die. One very important site of miliary spread is the meninges when tuberculous meningitis results.

The primary complex confers a measure of resistance to further infection, but this is by no means absolute and second infections do occur not uncommonly. The response to second infection is somewhat different to the primary infection. The inflammation induced is of a great degree and there is much more damage to the host tissues. The result is that there is a slowly expanding area of inflammation with death of the tissue in the centre. In tuberculosis the dead tissue has a characteristic 'cheesy' appearance and is described as being CASEOUS; the process is known as CASEATION. Surrounding the area of caseation is the characteristic inflammatory tissue of tuberculosis made up of many tubercles. This is the chronic granuloma of tuberculosis. There are often some areas in the inflammation which partially heal with the production of fibrous tissue. Tuberculosis at this stage is often known as FIBRO-CASEOUS tuberculosis. At this stage of the disease involving the lungs, tuberculous material may be coughed up, the patient then spreading the disease to other people. He is known as an 'open' case of pulmonary tuberculosis because tubercle bacilli can be detected in his sputum. A 'closed' case of tuberculosis does not have tubercle bacilli in the sputum; the disease process is not in direct contact with the air passages, and he cannot pass on his infection.

Secondary tuberculosis may involve organs other than the lungs. The kidneys may be the site of tuberculous inflammation when there will be a progressive destruction of these organs. The tubercle bacillus may be detected in the urine. Bones and joints are also not uncommonly involved.

Four main drugs are currently used in the treatment of tuberculosis. These are streptomycin by injection, isoniazid (INH), rifampicin and ethambutol by mouth. Most commonly three of these substances are given simultaneously as this has been found to reduce the rate at which the tubercle bacilli develop resistance to the drugs.

SYPHILIS

The causative organism of syphilis is the spirochaete *Treponema pallidum*. The disease is one of the venereal diseases, that is it is transferred from case to case by sexual contact. The spirochaete of syphilis is a very delicate organism, it dies quickly on removal from the body and on drying; it cannot be cultured in the laboratory. It is also difficult to stain, and is seen and identified by the use of a special type of microscopy known as DARK GROUND MICROSCOPY.

Syphilis is usually described as having three stages. After infection by contact with a sufferer from the disease there is a period of about three weeks during which nothing appears to happen. A red raised area then develops at the site of infection and later ulcerates. This is known as the PRIMARY CHANCRE. The most common site for a primary chancre is on the genitalia, but it may occur on the lips, tongue and rarely on the fingers. *T. pallidum* can be easily seen in the discharge from the ulcerated chancre using dark ground microscopy. The primary chancre is highly infectious, and contact with it is likely to result in transmission of the disease. Even if not treated the chancre will slowly heal and the patient may believe himself to be cured.

The SECONDARY STAGE of the disease usually starts a month or so after the appearance of the primary chancre. The patient is generally ill with headaches, chills and often vague aches and pains. He develops skin rashes, and ulcers occur in the mouth and on the genitals. The spirochaete has spread widely throughout the body and can be found easily in the discharges from the ulcers. These are again highly infectious to others. The secondary stage clears up spontaneously within a few weeks.

The TERTIARY STAGE does not usually start for several years. Chronic granulomata occur in various sites in the body. These differ from the inflammation of fibro-caseous tuberculosis in that there is very much more fibrous tissue and that although the centre of the inflammatory reaction dies, it does not become as soft and cheesy as tuberculous caseation. This inflammatory reaction is known as a GUMMA. Gummas are found in the liver, bones, genitalia, indeed they may occur anywhere. In some organs, notably the central nervous system and the cardiovascular system, the typical gumma is not seen and the inflammatory process is found diffusely through the tissues. Syphilis of the nervous system may produce a wide variety of clinical pictures. The commonest are tabes dorsalis, where the main damage is to the spinal cord, and general paralysis of the insane (GPI), where there is considerable brain damage. In the cardiovascular system the aorta and aortic valves are commonly affected, resulting in aortic incompetence and sometimes aneurism (dilatation) of the aorta.

In tertiary syphilis the spirochaetes are very scanty

and difficult to find. The diagnosis is made on the clinical findings and confirmed by the use of antibody tests. Tests commonly used include the Wassermann reaction and the VDRL (Venereal Diseases Reference Laboratory) test or some variation of it. These tests become positive just before or at the time of the secondary stage and are of great value in the diagnosis of the unusual skin rashes which occur in this stage. Unfortunately they may occasionally give positive reactions in diseases other than syphilis, 'false positive' reactions, and therefore positive reactions are usually confirmed with more specific tests such as the Treponema pallidum immobilisation test (TPI) and the absorbed fluorescent treponemal antibody test (FTA—ABS).

Penicillin in adequate dosage will kill *T. pallidum* and is successful in curing both the primary and secondary stages of the disease. If the disease has reached the tertiary stage the damage produced will still remain although the organisms will be destroyed.

Chapter Eleven

GENERALISED INFECTIONS

In some bacterial infections micro-organisms are to be found not only in one area of infection, but can be isolated from specimens taken from several or many sites in the body. Such infections are known as generalised infections. Spread of infection throughout the body may be the result of failure of the local body defences to contain an infection, or may invariably occur as a distinct phase in a specific infective disease. Micro-organisms spread in the body by means of two main routes—the blood and the lymph. Lymphatic spread is often arrested by an intervening lymph node, but if this fails, micro-organisms will pass eventually into the blood stream. Blood spread of infection is then ultimately the most important method and is usually divided into three types. From time to time in healthy individuals bacteria may enter the blood from which they are normally removed by the body defence mechanisms. This passive and transient presence of bacteria in the blood is known as BACTERAEMIA. If the body defences are inadequate so that the bacteria persist and multiply in the blood the condition is termed SEPTICAEMIA. If infective particles are spread by the blood and result in numerous secondary abscesses the condition is called PYAEMIA.

Bacteraemia literally means 'bacteria in the blood'

and is a surprisingly common occurrence in normal individuals. There is no general reaction to a few bacteria entering the blood stream; they are usually rapidly killed and the episode goes unnoticed. Bacteraemia certainly occurs after tooth extraction, chewing, and may even occur without any obvious precipitating cause. As already mentioned, bacteraemia usually does not result in disease, but on occasions the bacteria may settle in a suitable site for multiplication and an infection results. It is in this way that bacteria reach the heart valves to cause infection there (bacterial endocarditis), and may be the means whereby bacteria reach an internal structure, there to cause an infection. Diseases such as osteomyelitis (infection of a bone) may arise in this way. Spread is by means of the blood stream in many diseases caused by viruses. In virus infections the condition is known as VIRAEMIA. In the common diseases of childhood, measles and chickenpox, the generalised nature of the disease is due to blood spread after the virus has entered and established itself in the body.

In septicaemia, which is a consequence of the failure of the local body defences to contain the bacterial attack, micro-organisms and their toxins reach the blood stream and are distributed around the body. They may settle in any organ in the body and here produce further inflammation. The body suffers generally from a severe toxaemia. Septicaemia may arise from a localised pyogenic infection such as an abscess or may be a phase of an infectious disease such as enteric fever or brucellosis. In such diseases, in which septicaemia is a normal part of the infectious process, the invading micro-organisms invariably overcome the local body defences at their portal of entry and spread throughout the body. In septicaemia the offending micro-organism may be isolated from the blood; this usually provides a very useful diagnostic test.

Pyaemia is a complication of a pyogenic infection. The name means literally 'pus in the blood'. The most important difference between pyaemia and septicaemia is in the size of the masses of bacteria entering the blood stream. In pyaemia these are relatively large clumps of bacteria and pus cells, whereas in septicaemia solitary bacteria are more usual. The effect of the large clumps of bacteria in pyaemia is to block small blood vessels, shutting off the blood supply to a small piece of tissue, thus reducing the local resistance to infection. The bacteria in the clump find themselves in an ideal site for multiplication, and an abscess results. Multiple PYAEMIC ABSCESSES in various organs are the usual and characteristic finding of pyaemia.

In order to illustrate the spread of micro-organisms in generalised infections several different diseases will be considered. These are enteric fever, brucellosis, subacute bacterial endocarditis, plague and measles.

ENTERIC FEVER is the name given to a group of diseases caused by several bacteria of the genus *Salmonella*. These are *Salm. typhi*, *Salm. paratyphi A*, *Salm. paratyphi B* and *Salm. paratyphi C*. Alternatively enteric fever may be named TYPHOID or PARATYPHOID. The causative organism of enteric fever enters the body by the mouth, carried there in food or water which has been contaminated by a case or carrier of the disease. The bacteria pass through the wall of the intestine and settle to multiply in various organs. The liver, the spleen and lymphoid tissue are the main sites of multiplication. This process takes about two weeks and is followed by passage of the bacteria and toxins into the blood with general symptoms of septicaemia. This is the clinical onset of the disease: the initial multiplication having taken place without serious upset to the patient. Bacteria may be isolated from the blood during this stage of the disease, and also usually from the urine, which they reach after being filtered from the blood by the kidneys. At this stage of the disease the patient presents with a temperature (pyrexia) and general toxaemia, but with little else to indicate the nature of the disease. It is an important cause of PYREXIA OF UNKNOWN ORIGIN (PUO). Later the bacteria invade and multiply in the lymphoid tissue of the intestine and now may be isolated more easily from the faeces. Contrary to popular belief, the bacteria can be isolated from the faeces in the first week in only about half of the cases. The test for antibodies to the causative organisms is called the WIDAL TEST and may be used to assist in making the diagnosis. Ulceration, haemorrhage and perforation may result from the attack on the intestine. The antibiotic of choice for the treatment of enteric fever is chloramphenicol. Other drugs which have been used with variable success are ampicillin and co-trimoxazole.

BRUCELLOSIS is a subacute or chronic disease caused by bacteria of the genus *Brucella*. The disease presents as an intermittent pyrexia which continues for months and is associated with a general feeling of ill-health. The disease reaches man in milk from diseased cattle, and in areas in which goats' milk is used, from infected goats. After entry into the body the bacteria multiply mainly in the lymphoid tissue. They appear to be able to survive and to multiply inside the larger cells of the lymphoid tissue. *Brucella* may also enter the blood and can be isolated from this site. The septicaemia of brucellosis is intermittent and the number of bacteria in the blood is less than in most other septicaemic conditions, both factors making the isolation of the organism difficult. Diagnosis is confirmed by culture of the blood on repeated occasions, and by antibody tests.

SUBACUTE BACTERIAL ENDOCARDITIS (SABE) is an infection involving the lining of the heart (endocardium), mostly commonly that covering the heart valves. The most common causative organism is *Streptococcus viridans* which is a normal inhabitant of the upper respiratory tract. Other bacteria including other streptococci may cause the disease and *Staphylococcus aureus* causes acute disease. The infection starts on a valve previously damaged by rheumatic heart disease, but may also occur on a part of the endocardium which is abnormal because of a congenital malformation. *Strept. viridans* reaches the damaged valve during the transient bacteraemia which not uncommonly occurs in normal individuals, and which certainly takes place during dental manipulations. A small plug of fibrin develops on the infected endocardium, and this is known as a VEGETATION. Small vegetations may break off the endocardium and pass via the blood stream to other organs, there producing further tissue damage. *Strept. viridans* may be isolated by blood culture. Treatment is difficult because the body defences are hampered by the lack of an efficient inflammatory response. Penicillin in high dosage for a long period of time sometimes with gentamicin is the usual method of treatment when *Strep. viridans* is the causative organism. Prophylactic treatment with penicillin is often given before dental operations in individuals with rheumatic or congenital heart disease, to prevent the occurrence of SABE.

PLAGUE is a disease of considerable historical importance. Vast epidemics of the disease have killed millions of people. The disease is now fortunately rare in civilised communities, but is still to be found in under-developed countries. The causative organism is the Gram-negative bacillus *Pasteurella pestis*. The disease occurs in rats and is spread amongst the rat population by the rat flea. When a rat dies of plague the fleas search for a new host and if a further rat is not available will attack man. The flea implants the plague bacilli into the skin of man either directly during the biting or indirectly by contaminating the skin with faeces containing the micro-organism which, because of the itching produced, are scratched into the skin. After an incubaton period of about a week during which multiplication of the bacteria takes place, the local lymph nodes become painful and swollen. The enlarged, inflamed lymph nodes are known as 'buboes' and the disease is often called BUBONIC PLAGUE for this reason. This localised inflammation may be followed by septicaemia with sometimes coma. The organism may be isolated from the blood and from any tissue during this stage. Bleeding into the skin often occurs, producing discoloured areas which gave the disease its old name of 'the black death'. Once septicaemia has occurred the death rate even with treatment is high. The disease may spread from man to man by droplet infection during an epidemic; the portal of entry is now the lungs and an even more severe form of the disease is found—PNEUMONIC PLAGUE.

MEASLES is a common disease of childhood characterised by fever, cough, a skin rash, nasal discharge and inflammation of the conjunctiva. It is caused by a virus, and probably spread by droplet infection from child to child. Although usually in itself a mild disease, it lowers the body resistance to other infections which often occur as a complication of measles. When measles is introduced into a population in which it does not normally occur, i.e. an isolated group of people, the disease itself can be of considerable severity. The incubation period of the disease is about 14 days, during which it is presumed that the virus multiplies in the body, possibly in lymphoid tissue, without producing symptoms. The virus then spreads throughout the body by way of the blood. The characteristic symptoms of measles occur at this time. The disease is rapidly overcome by the body defences without the necessity for treatment although any complications occurring must be detected and treated.

It will be seen that there is a general pattern of behaviour in the diseases in which general spread of infection is the rule. The relationship of the invader to the host is such that initially the body defences are overcome; multiplication takes place and is then followed by spread throughout the body. After this the body wins the battle, possibly requiring assistance in the form of medical treatment, or the patient dies. The type of micro-organism which produces this type of disease is very well adapted to the pathogenic existence; it either has very good weapons of attack which overcome the initial attempts to remove it or is not initially susceptible to the body defences, as in the case of measles virus and *Brucella*, by being able to live and multiply inside the cells of the body.

Chapter Twelve

INFECTIONS OF THE
RESPIRATORY TRACT

The respiratory tract may be divided for the purpose of this chapter into the UPPER RESPIRATORY TRACT comprising the nose and nasal passages, the mouth, the pharynx and the larynx, and the LOWER RESPIRAT-ORY TRACT being the trachea, the bronchi and the lungs. The airway has thus been divided into two above and below the larynx. Acute infections of the two areas are considered separately.

UPPER RESPIRATORY TRACT INFECTIONS

To be considered under this heading are the two very important infections of the fauces and pharynx caused by *Corynebacterium diphtheriae* and by *Streptococcus pyogenes*, together with the less important infections, Vincent's angina and the virus infections of the upper respiratory tract.

DIPHTHERIA is a disease in which there is a local infection, usually in the pharynx, but which may also extend further into the respiratory tract or occur in the nose. This is associated with the production of a toxin which can cause very serious damage to other organs. The causative organism is *Corynebacterium diphtheriae* and the toxin is known as diphtheria toxin. Of recent years the disease has been uncommon in communities with efficient medical services because of prophylactic immunisation, but it still occurs from time to time and is also a not inconsiderable problem in countries in which an immunisation programme has not been carried out.

The local infection in the nose or throat will be noticed as a nasal discharge or as a severe 'sore throat'. There is a pyogenic reaction in the infected tissue, but in addition the effect of the diphtheria toxin is to kill the tissue cells locally, producing a grey, dead-looking area of tissue. This is described as a MEMBRANE. The inflammation may spread down the respiratory tract where it may cause obstruction of the airway, particularly if it involves the larynx. Diphtheria toxin is absorbed from the local infection and is distributed throughout the body. It produces severe damage to the heart muscle and to nervous tissue causing difficulty in swallowing and breathing. The effects of the toxin may cause death of the patient. Treatment is directed towards neutralising the toxin by the use of injections of diphtheria antitoxin prepared in horses. If given early in the course of the disease this method of treatment is effective, but once the diphtheria toxin has combined with the target tissues the tissue damage is not reversible. Penicillin and erythromycin are effective in killing *C. diphtheriae*, but antibiotic treatment is less important than antitoxin treatment.

STREPTOCOCCUS PYOGENES INFECTIONS of the upper respiratory tract usually involve the tonsils but may spread to nearby tissues in the pharynx. The organism is a Gram-positive coccus which occurs in chains. Streptococci are divided up into large groups according to the type of lysis which they produce when grown on media containing red blood cells (blood agar). The streptococci of most importance in medicine are those which produce an area of complete clearing of the red cells around a colony. This is known as BETA-HAEMOLYSIS, and such streptococci are known as beta-haemolytic streptococci. Other streptococci produce a green colour in the area of haemolysis around a colony—ALPHA-HAEMOLYSIS; these are known as *Strept. viridans*. Many streptococci produce no haemolysis—non-haemolytic streptococci. *Strept. pyogenes* is a beta-haemolytic streptococcus of a type known as Lancefield group A. The Lancefield group of a streptococcus is determined by a serological technique, and group A is by far the most important.

Streptococcal tonsillitis is a common infection which presents as a sore throat and fever often with considerable general aches and pains in the limbs. The patient is often considerably more ill than the local infection in the throat would suggest he should be. There is a pyogenic reaction in the infected area with redness and swelling and often pus is visible on the surface of the tonsil. Some strains of *Strept. pyogenes* produce a toxin which damages the skin, giving rise to a rash. This is the ERYTHROGENIC TOXIN, and the disease is known as SCARLATINA or SCARLET FEVER if the rash occurs. Apart from the skin rash, which is of minor inconvenience only, there is no difference between a *Strept. pyogenes* tonsillitis and scarlatina. Antibody is formed against the erythrogenic toxin and so even though one may have many attacks of streptococcal tonsillitis the rash of scarlet fever usually only occurs during the first attack. The condition is cured rapidly by penicillin, to which antibiotic the organism is very sensitive.

Two important complications may occur after

infection with *Strept. pyogenes*. These are rheumatic fever and nephritis. Two to four weeks after recovery from a *Strept. pyogenes* infection the patient may develop evidence of damage either to the kidneys (nephritis) or to the joints and heart (rheumatic fever). Actual infection of the kidneys, heart and joints with the streptococci is not the cause and a form of hyper-sensitivity reaction to the infecting streptococci is the explanation. It is significant that in rheumatic fever antibodies develop to streptococcal antigens which are similar to human heart muscle antigens. In acute strep-tococcal infection every effort must be made to eradi-cate the streptococci and thus eliminate the antigenic stimulus.

VINCENT'S ANGINA is a disease which causes ulcera-tion in the mouth and sometimes in the pharynx. It is caused by two micro-organisms which are found together in the inflammatory exudate. These are a long thin spirochaete—*Borrelia vincenti*, and a Gram-negative bacillus—*Fusobacterium fusiforme*. The ulcers formed are shallow and the condition is often associ-ated with a poor standard of dental hygiene. The diag-nosis is made entirely on the examination of a stained smear of the exudate when both types of organism are are seen in large numbers. Treatment consists of cor-recting the dental condition and the administration of penicillin or metronidazole.

VIRUS INFECTIONS OF THE UPPER RESPIRATORY TRACT are very common indeed. We all suffer from time to time from conditions called common colds. In fact quite a large variety of viruses produce the symptoms which we associate with the common cold—pyrexia, nasal discharge, headaches, sore throat. The true cold viruses have been isolated, but in addition the *adenoviruses*, the *coxsackie viruses*, the ECHO viruses, *parainfleunza viruses*, and others are isolated from conditions which often would be described as 'a cold'. Other symptoms may sometimes suggest which virus is involved. Thus adenoviruses may commonly cause a sore throat, coxsackie infections may result in ulceration of the pharynx, whilst parainfluenza infections may have croup as the main symptom. It is however impossible to make an accurate clinical diagnosis of the virus involved, and the amount of work and time required to isolate and identify these viruses is considerable.

LOWER RESPIRATORY TRACT INFECTIONS

Infections of the lower respiratory tract include chronic and acute bronchitis, pneumonia, which will be considered under the headings bronchopneumonia, lobar pneumonia and atypical pneumonia, and whooping cough.

CHRONIC BRONCHITIS is a very common disease in this country. It is characterised by a chronic cough which produces thick viscid sputum. The primary cause is almost certainly not bacterial, and atmospheric pollution, smoking, and in some cases allergy to environmental antigens, are more likely causative factors. Bacteria however play a part in maintaining and causing deterioration of the condition. Sufferers from chronic bronchitis tend to develop episodes of acute infection which occur most commonly in the winter months, and are often preceded by a virus upper respiratory tract infection. Repeated episodes of acute infection tend to damage still further the already diseased bronchi and lungs, and heart failure may eventually occur.

The organism most commonly isolated from the sputum during acute episodes in sufferers from chronic bronchitis is *Haemophilus influenzae*; others include pneumococci, staphylococci and coliforms. The avoidance of acute episodes is of such importance that many physicians treat the patient with antibiotics for the whole of the winter months in the hope of preventing acute bacterial infections. Another method is to give the patient a supply of antibiotic with the suggestion that he take it if he develops a cold or the weather is foggy. Antibiotics most often used for this purpose are tetracycline and ampicillin.

ACUTE BRONCHITIS usually occurs in normal individuals as a complication of an upper respiratory tract infection. Instead of the expected rapid recovery, the patient develops a cough with purulent sputum. The illness is not so severe as that found in acute infection in chronic bronchitis and responds well to treatment with antibiotics. The same types of bacteria are found in the sputum as those described as occurring in acute episodes of chronic bronchitis.

BRONCHOPNEUMONIA is an infection of the lungs. It is best considered as an extension of acute bronchitis. The inflammatory process has spread beyond the bronchi to involve the bronchioles and the alveoli of the lung. The disease is much more serious and may be fatal. The normal individual rarely develops bronchopneumonia as a complication of acute bronchitis, but this may occur in the young child, in an old person, and in persons of all ages who for some reason have a decreased resistance to infection. This is often found after anaesthesia, and many of the patients with 'a post-operative chest' have mild bronchopneumonia, often associated with small areas of pulmonary collapse. In addition, the damage caused in the respiratory tract by virus infections such as influenza will predispose to bronchopneumonia. Because of the route by which infection reaches the lung, i.e. via the bronchi, the inflammation in the lung is patchy. Areas of pyogenic inflammatory exudate are found around small bronchi and bronchioles. Inflammatory exudate in the alveoli of the lung gives the tissue a solid feel, known as CONSOLIDATION. Thus bronchopneumonia results in patchy areas of consolidation in relation to bronchi and bronchioles. The organisms which cause bronchopneumonia include the pneumococcus, *Haemophilis influenzae*, *Staphylococcus aureus*, coliforms and others. Antibiotic treatment of choice is determined by laboratory testing of the organism isolated from sputum.

LOBAR PNEUMONIA is so named because the inflammation is often of a whole lobe of the lung. This is unlike bronchopneumonia where the inflammation is patchy. Lobar pneumonia is an acute disease which affects all age groups and is not limited to the young and the old. The causative organism is the pneumococcus. The pneumococcus has a slimy capsule which prevents the ingestion of the organism by phagocytes; in the first stages of infection the organism is therefore not restricted. Spread is also encouraged by the outpouring of fluid into the alveoli. The lobe of the lung becomes firm and airless as a result of the cellular and fluid exudate; it is consolidated. Spread to other lobes may occur but is not common because the fibrous tissue between the lobes acts as a barrier. If the patient does not die of overwhelming infection and toxaemia in the earlier stages of the disease, antibody is eventually formed. The most important antibody is that directed against the antigens in the bacterial capsule. Once antibody has stuck onto the capsule of the pneumococcus, phagocytosis may proceed normally. With the body defences now able to cope efficiently with the invader the disease process is rapidly brought under control. Clinically this rapid improvement in the situation is seen as a fall in temperature with recovery of the patient. This is known as resolution by 'crisis'. Some cases of pneumonia may recover more slowly—resolution by 'lysis'.

The pneumococcus is usually very sensitive to penicillin, and as this antibiotic is usually given to the patient in the early stages of the disease, the inflammation subsides without reaching the stage of extensive consolidation and without a 'crisis'. Indeed, the typical established clinical picture of lobar pneumonia is now rarely seen.

ATYPICAL PNEUMONIA was a term first used in the mid thirties when 'typical' pneumonia was that caused by the pneumococcus or haemolytic streptococcus. It was atypical in that no causative bacteria could be isolated from the sputum, the symptoms were general rather than respiratory and that x-rays of the chest showed more extensive disease than the patient's symptoms suggested. The commonest and most important cause is *Mycoplasma pneumoniae*, an organism similar to bacteria, but having no cell-wall. With special techniques it can be isolated from the sputum, but the diagnosis usually depends on the demonstration of antibodies. Other causes include Q fever and psittacosis (Ch. Fifteen). Atypical pneumonia caused by *M. pneumoniae* is most usually treated with one of the tetracycline group of antibiotics. Several viruses including the influenza and parainfluenza viruses and adenovirus may cause pneumonia.

WHOOPING COUGH (pertussis) is a common disease of childhood caused by *Bordetella pertussis*. Clinically the child often suffers initially from symptoms of an upper respiratory tract infection, but later develops a persistent cough. In typical cases the 'whoop' is heard. This is a noisy, high pitched inspiration following a series of coughs when most of the air is expelled from the child's lung due to difficulty in coughing up thick sputum. Often a typical 'whoop' does not occur or is missed. Vomiting after coughing is a symptom which occurs in whooping cough, particularly in small children. The post-nasal space is the best site from which to isolate *Bord. pertussis*. Specimens are obtained either using an approach through the mouth with a West's swab or through the nose using a per-nasal swab. The organism dies rapidly if not placed on suitable media. An alternative method is to take a COUGH PLATE. A Petri dish of suitable medium is placed a few inches in front of the child's mouth as it coughs. This is then incubated. Patience may be required in waiting for a suitably explosive cough and anyone collecting the specimen can protect themselves by holding a piece of clear x-ray film between their face and the patient. The majority of patients recover spontaneously, but whooping cough is never a trivial disease. In some cases it results in permanent lung damage, and death can occur, particularly in children under one year of age. Antibiotics are rarely of any value once the disease is established, but they can be given to healthy contacts to prevent them contracting the illness and erythromycin and co-trimoxazole have been used for this purpose. Skilled calm and reassuring nursing is probably the most important aspect of treatment of the often terrified patient. Vaccination can certainly reduce the rate of attack and the severity of the illness when it occurs in vaccinated children. However, batches of vaccine can vary in potency and effectiveness and complications of vaccination may rarely include convulsions, paralysis and mental retardation.

Chapter Thirteen

INFECTIONS OF THE
GASTRO-INTESTINAL TRACT

Infections of the gastro-intestinal tract are very common. They vary in severity from mild diarrhoea to severe and sometimes fatal cholera. Gastro-intestinal infections are most common and tend to be most severe in tropical countries. In this country gastro-intestinal infections are most common during the summer months. Diarrhoea and vomiting are the two important symptoms of gastro-intestinal infection, but only one or other of the two symptoms may be present in a particular case. Most infections of the gastro-intestinal tract are spread by means of contaminated food or drink. The contamination reaches the food from infected cases or animals directly, or may be transferred from infected excreta by insects, e.g. flies. Any case of food-borne infection indicates a failure in food hygiene, and as such requires correction if more persons are not to become infected. Having isolated a pathogenic organism from a case of gastro-intestinal infection we must attempt to discover the source of infection and remove it. Most of this 'detective' work is carried out by the Environmental Health Authorities, who will be notified of cases of infection by the medical practitioner attending the patient. Often it is not possible to discover the source of infection in a single case, but when several or many persons are infected the chances of finding the source increase.

The diseases which are considered in this chapter are bacillary dysentery, 'food poisoning', gastro-enteritis of children, and cholera.

BACILLARY DYSENTERY is an infection of the gastro-intestinal tract with bacilli of the genus *Shigella*. It is more common in children than adults. The principal symptom of this disease is diarrhoea which may be mild or severe. If severe the faeces are liquid and contain mucus and often blood. The patient will have a raised temperature and will have general symptoms of toxaemia. There are several species of *Shigella* which cause dysentery, *Sh. sonnei* causes a relatively mild form of the disease, *Sh. flexneri* and *Sh. dysenteriae* producing a much more severe illness, the last in tropical countries. Unlike the other diseases described in this chapter, Sonne dysentery, which is by far the most common type in Great Britain, is now not often spread by contaminated food and is more common in the winter than the summer. Although the organisms may be taken in with food they are usually spread by direct person to person contact or by inanimate objects such as toys or towels. The picture of dysentery has not always been one of a mild sporadic disease of children. In the past it has ravaged armies and today in tropical countries with poor standards of hygiene it can still be responsible for large food- or water-borne outbreaks of disease. Diagnosis is confirmed by isolating the organism from the faeces. Selective media are used which suppress the growth of many of the faecal organisms, but which allow *Shigella* and other pathogens to grow. Treatment is directed towards control of the diarrhoea with simple mixtures such as those containing Kaolin. Antibiotics are used only in severe cases and then they must be chosen with the help of sensitivity tests since resistance is a serious problem. Even if they do eliminate the organism from the faeces, which they do not always do, there is some doubt about whether they change the course of the disease and in mild forms they certainly do not.

FOOD POISONING is a name for the gastro-intestinal upsets which are associated with eating contaminated food. It is not a single condition and there are several possible causes for an outbreak of food poisoning. The typical story of an outbreak of food poisoning is that a group of persons become ill with evidence of gastro-intestinal irritation after eating a meal together. The cause may not be bacterial; excessive eating and drinking can in itself cause diarrhoea and vomiting. Again, irritant substances might have found their way into the food by accident. The causes of bacterial food poisoning are of two types. The first is due to the presence in the food of pre-formed bacterial toxin and the second type is due to bacterial infection usually with organisms of the genus *Salmonella* or *Campylobacter*.

Toxin may be produced in food if it is first contaminated with bacteria and then stored under unsuitable conditions for some time. During the storage period the bacteria grow and produce the toxin. The two micro-organisms which are most commonly implicated in pre-formed toxin food poisoning are *Staphylococcus aureus* and *Clostridium perfringens* (*welchii*). The type of food often involved is cooked meat which is either served cold or reheated. After cooking the food is allowed to cool slowly or it is subsequently warmed. The food is thus allowed to remain for some time at temperatures which permit bacteria to multiply and produce toxin. Once the toxin has been

formed heating will not destroy it. Food which is
thoroughly cooked and served hot without storage is
safe. Storage of cooked foods must be carried out
under conditions in which bacterial growth cannot
take place. Refrigeration is a suitable method. Contamination of the food can sometimes be traced
directly to one of the food handlers.

Staphylococcal infections of the skin such as
infected cuts or boils is a common source of *Staph.
aureus* contamination of food. Ideally, food handlers
with such infections should be given another job until
the infection has cleared. The symptoms of pre-
formed toxin food poisoning start soon after eating the
contaminated food, from half an hour to five hours
with the *Staphylococcus* and usually between 12 and 24
hours with *Clostridium perfringens*. Abdominal pain is
very common, particularly with the clostridial type
of disease, and the patient may suffer from general
toxaemia sometime associated with considerable
shock. Vomiting is the predominant feature of the
staphylococcal disease. The course of the illness is
short and recovery is usually complete within a day.

A rare but interesting form of food poisoning
caused by a bacterial toxin is botulism which is caused
by the toxin produced by *Clostridium botulinum*. The
poison is one of the most powerful known and as little
as twelve millionths of a gram will kill a man. The
disease is usually caused by home canned or home
boiled foods which are not heated enough to kill the
spore-bearing organism. The symptoms include
severe weakness and paralysis with an inability to
swallow. It is often fatal.

Salmonellas may reach food from several sources.
They may be inadvertently placed there by a food

handler who is suffering from the infection himself, or who has recently recovered from infection and is still excreting *Salmonella*. The food may be contaminated with animal excreta containing *Salmonella*; rats and mice are probably the worst offenders. The animal providing the source of food may have been infected at the time it was killed. This is especially the case in poultry. If the food is thoroughly cooked and served immediately there is no risk of infection because the organisms will be killed. Uncooked foods, and foods which are stored provide the usual source of infection.

There are many species in the genus *Salmonella*: these are identified by the use of specific antibodies. Two commonly involved in food poisoning in this country are *Salm. typhi-murium*, which is a natural pathogen of mice, and *Salm. enteritidis*. It should be noted that the organisms of enteric fever belong to the genus *Salmonella*, but that the species which cause Salmonella food poisoning do not cause enteric fever and *vice versa*. The two diseases are quite distinct from each other even though the causative organisms belong to the same genus.

The symptoms of Salmonella food poisoning include diarrhoea, abdominal discomfort, pyrexia and sometimes vomiting. The symptoms do not start as soon after eating the contaminated food as do those of pre-formed toxin food poisoning, there being an interval of about 24 hours between infection and symptoms. The symptoms subside in a few days, even without antibiotic treatment, but the organisms may persist in the faeces for weeks or even longer. There is no septicaemic phase as in enteric fever. Diagnosis is confirmed by isolating the organism from the faeces and if available from vomitus and from suspect food.

It has recently been shown that a common cause of food poisoning, perhaps the most common cause, is *Campylobacter jejunalis*. This microaerophilic organism grows best at 43°C. Infection may be acquired from other cases or carriers or from food and drink such as milk, poultry and pork, or even from sick domestic animals such as a dog. If food is cooked it is rendered safe since this kills the organisms. The interval between infection and symptoms is about two to ten days. The symptoms include diarrhoea and, less commonly, vomiting and abdominal pain. The antibiotic which has been used with most success seems to be erythromycin.

GASTRO-ENTERITIS OF CHILDREN is an important disease of early life which carries a not inconsiderable mortality. The child, usually a few months old, suffers from severe vomiting and diarrhoea and may die of dehydration if not treated rapidly. Some cases are due to *Salmonella* infection, but the most important group of cases are caused by several strains of *Escherichia coli*. This organism is a normal inhibitant of the intestine, but some strains—ENTERO-PATHOGENIC STRAINS, are able to cause infection in the very young. These are in many respects very similar to the common inhabitants of the intestine and they can only be identified by antibody typing. Infection is spread by poor hygiene, particularly failure to sterilise feeding utensils. The source of infection is probably symptom-free adults or other children. Diagnosis is confirmed by isolating the organism from the faeces. The organism may be sensitive to tetracyclines, neomycin and chloramphenicol which have all been used in the treatment. Of paramount importance in the treatment is the correction of dehydration by means of intravenous fluids.

CHOLERA is a tropical disease caused by the organism *Vibrio cholera*. It is most common in the Far East, where large epidemics have occurred in the past, and still occur from time to time. The infection is usually spread by means of unsatisfactory drinking water which is contaminated by a human sufferer from the disease. Adequately purified, i.e. filtered or chlorinated, water is safe. The symptoms of cholera start about one or two days after drinking contaminated water. They are caused by a toxin produced by the organism which acts on the lining or mucosa of the intestine causing it to pour out fluid. Profuse diarrhoea with 'rice water' stools follows with pyrexia, abdominal pain and general toxaemia. The patient may die of dehydration and the mortality rate may be as high as 80%. The organism may be isolated from the faeces although sometimes this is only achieved with difficulty. Vaccines are available for protection against cholera, but repeat doses should be given at about six monthly intervals to maintain immunity. The most important part of treatment is replacement of lost fluid and electrolytes by intravenous therapy. Many antibiotics will kill the organism, but tetracycline is particularly effective in reducing fluid loss.

Chapter Fourteen

INFECTIONS OF THE NERVOUS SYSTEM

Infection of the central nervous system (CNS) may involve the meninges when it is known as MENINGITIS, the brain, ENCEPHALITIS, or the spinal cord, MYELITIS. If both the brain and the spinal cord are involved it is known as ENCEPHALOMYELITIS and if both the meninges and brain are affected it is called MENINGO-ENCEPHALITIS. Infections may be caused by bacteria viruses or fungi.

BACTERIAL MENINGITIS has already been discussed (p. 82) and separate mention has been made of tuberculous meningitis (p. 92). In the latter condition most of the cells found on examination of the cerebrospinal fluid (c.s.f.) are lymphocytes whereas in meningitis caused by other bacteria the majority of cells are polymorphonuclear leucocytes, 'polymorphs'.

In VIRAL MENINGITIS most of the cells found in the c.s.f. are lymphocytes, but the c.s.f. glucose concentration is usually normal unlike the situation in tuberculous meningitis in which the c.s.f. glucose is reduced. The viruses most commonly associated with meningitis or meningoencephalitis in Britain are MUMPS, HERPES SIMPLEX, COXSACKIE and ECHO. A sudden onset of headache and fever is the usual way in which the illness starts with all the viruses. If there is ENCEPHALITIS the patient may become drowsy or go into a coma and the patient may have a behavioural disturbance or become confused particularly with *Herpes simplex*. There may be other evidence of damage to the brain such as convulsions, tremor, abnormalities of eye co-ordination or facial palsy. Serological tests may help in making the diagnosis by demonstrating a rise in antibodies to one of the viruses and virus culture may also be successful. However, it is not always possible to grow a virus from the c.s.f. and although one may be shown to be present in the faeces or the throat, the results of these tests are usually available too late to guide treatment. It is not yet clear whether or not antiviral drugs help in the treatment of these diseases but IDOXURIDINE and CYTARABINE have been used in the treatment of herpes encephalitis.

Outside Britain encephalitis may be caused by viruses which are transmitted to man by the bite of arthropods and insects such as mosquitos and ticks. The arthropod borne viruses, ARBOVIRUSES, may cause epidemics of encephalitis which have been well studied. Examples are Eastern and Western encephalitis and Venezuelan equine encephalitis.

RABIES is a form of encephalitis which is always fatal and due to a virus which infects a wide variety of animals including dogs, cats and foxes. The virus is present in the saliva of infected animals and is transmitted to man by a bite usually from a dog. The virus spreads from the wound to the CNS via the nerves. The symptoms consist of excitement, muscular contractions, convulsions and spasm of the muscles of swallowing, hence the older name for the disease HYDROPHOBIA or fear of water. The diagnosis may be made most rapidly by direct demonstration of the virus in specimens such as the hair-bearing skin at the back of the neck, corneal impression smears or brain tissue.

Bacterial infections of the brain are pyogenic in nature, and usually take the form of abscesses. Bacteria may reach the brain in the blood stream as part of a septicaemia or pyaemia or may extend inwards from an infection outside the CNS. The commonest example of the latter type of spread is extension of a middle ear infection through the skull into the temporal lobe of the brain. Apart from the serious results of damage to a part of the nervous system, such abscesses are very similar to those already described in Chapter Nine, and they will not be discussed further.

POLIOMYELITIS is an acute virus disease in which the major damage is to the motor cells in the anterior horns of the spinal cord (Fig. 15). This results in an interruption in the pathway of the nervous control of muscle movement. The result is muscle weakness and paralysis. The degree of paralysis produced depends on the number and distribution of motor cells destroyed and damaged, and varies from weakness of one limb to complete paralysis of all four limbs, paralysis of the respiratory muscles, and often death. The disease attacks all age groups, but is usually most severe in adults.

For part of the life history of the virus, the cells lining the alimentary tract are infected and the virus may be detected in the faeces. In addition it may be isolated from the pharynx on occasions. The faeces and possibly the saliva are the vehicles by which the virus passes from case to case. Having infected the cells of the intestine, often without producing any symptoms, the disease process may cease and the person suffers no ill-effects. This type of subclinical infection

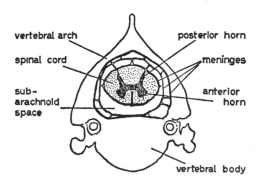

Fig. 15. Transverse section of a vertebra to show the structure of the spinal cord and meninges.

is relatively common, especially in a community in which the virus is widespread and the standards of hygiene are low. Under these circumstances many persons are infected, but few suffer from symptoms of the disease because they become infected in childhood when the nervous system seems to be more resistant to infection, or as a baby whilst still having a measure of passive immunity derived from the mother (see p. 44). If the infection does not remain subclinical viraemia occurs. The virus may be detected in the blood, and the patient suffers from a vague general illness with a raised temperature. The virus soon settles in the anterior horn cells of the spinal cord, and symptoms of muscle weakness and paralysis are produced. No anti- biotics will attack the polio virus, and treatment is directed towards preventing pyogenic infection and pneumonia, reducing the effects of paralysis by com- plete rest, and preventing the development of muscle contractions by maintaining the paralysed limbs in a suitable position. If the respiratory muscles are involved a ventilator is necessary to carry out breathing movements for the patient. If the patient survives the acute phase of the disease, some degree of recovery of muscle power can be expected. The amount of recovery varies from patient to patient.

Vaccines are available which give a considerable degree of protection against poliomyelitis. These are of two types—the SALK VACCINE which consists of killed polio virus of the three main strains, and SABIN VACCINE which consists of live virus which has been attenuated, i.e. is unable to cause damage to the CNS. The Salk vaccine is given by injection whereas the Sabin vaccine is given by mouth, when a subclinical infection with safe virus takes place. Three doses of vaccine are usually given.

HERPES ZOSTER, better simply called ZOSTER, is a disease of adults which is caused by the same virus which causes chickenpox in children. It is due to reactivation of the virus, lying dormant in the patient, many years after an attack of chickenpox. The fact that the adult may have himself suffered from chickenpox in childhood does not provide protection against the development of zoster. The disease presents as a painful and irritating rash on the skin in the distribution of one or more sensory nerves. The commonest site is in the distribution of the cutaneous nerves derived from the thoracic spinal cord. The rash passes obliquely around one side of the chest, being higher at the back than the front. The rash is made up of small blisters with surrounding redness. The virus can be isolated from the blisters, but the major damage is in the sensory ganglion on the posterior root of the spinal cord. The disease may involve cranial sensory nerves in addition to spinal nerves. Recovery is usually completed without any treatment, but secondary infection of the skin rash may occur, and in some patients the pain may persist for long periods and prove difficult to relieve.

Chapter Fifteen

VIRUSES CHLAMYDIAE AND
RICKETTSIAE

Not all micro-organisms of medical importance are bacteria. There are in addition the fungi and the protozoa, the latter being discussed in Chapter Sixteen, and the VIRUSES CHLAMYDIAE and RICKETTSIAE.

THE VIRUSES

The viruses differ from other micro-organisms in three important respects. First they are much smaller than bacteria varying in size from 0.01μ to 0.3μ, secondly they contain only one nucleic acid, DNA or RNA, whereas other organisms contain both, and thirdly, they cannot multiply outside living host cells. They consist of a central core of nucleic acid surrounded by a protein coat and they reproduce by invading a cell and redirecting it to produce virus particles. They are killed by heat and by some but not all of the disinfectants which kill bacteria. Both antibodies and cell-mediated immunity assist in protecting the body against virus infections, and in addition during the acute phase of a virus infection the infected cells release INTERFERON into the blood and tissues. This substance renders other cells resistant to virus infection.

Special methods are used in the diagnosis of virus disease. Viruses being very small cannot be seen with the normal light microscope. However, the direct demonstration of viruses is possible. They may be seen with an electron microscope, but this instrument is large and expensive and is not available in most hospital laboratories. Viruses may also be demonstrated by means of fluorescence. Antibodies to viruses can be made to fluoresce and attached to the antigens, the viruses in tissues. The fluorescent material can then be seen under a modified light microscope.

Viruses may also be grown, but only inside cells. Body secretions or other material for examination is best kept cool and in a special transport medium until it reaches the laboratory. The systems for providing the living cells in which the viruses may be grown are TISSUE CULTURE, CHICK EMBRYO and LABORATORY ANIMALS. Tissue culture is the system that is most commonly used. Cells from man or animals are grown in a single layer, MONOLAYER, on the walls of test tubes or on one side of flat bottles which contain a suitable solution into which the material for culture is placed. The bottles or tubes are incubated and after a few days the presence of the virus may be recognised by the degeneration or death of the cells of the culture. Occasionally viruses may grow in tissue culture without producing a visible change in the cells and their presence must be demonstrated by another method such as fluorescence.

Fertile hens' eggs contain living CHICK EMBRYOS. The eggs contain several cavities and membranes capable of supporting the growth of viruses. However, chick embryos are not capable of growing as many viruses as tissue cultures and now are less frequently used.

Some viruses will not grow in either fertile hens'

eggs or tissue cultures, but only in laboratory animals which, after inoculation, are observed for signs of disease or death.

Serology may also be used in the diagnosis of virus disease (p. 48). Samples of blood are taken from the patient in the acute phase of the illness and 14 days later, and a rise in the amount of antibodies to a particular virus demonstrated. This method of diagnosis is only possible if the number of viruses capable of causing the disease is limited. If the number is high then the number of tests required becomes excessive. The tests most usually employed to determine the amount of antibodies are known as COMPLEMENT FIXATION TESTS which are based upon the fact that when antibodies and antigens combine, COMPLEMENT, which is a complex constituent of human and animal serum, is 'fixed' or used up.

Some of the virus diseases of the CNS are described in Chapter Fourteen. Other characteristic virus diseases will now be discussed briefly, including influenza, some respiratory infections, hepatitis, mumps, measles and german measles.

The characteristic features of influenza are well known. They consist of fever, headache, generalised aches and sometimes a runny nose. The patient may have a cough and sore throat, and in severe cases pneumonia may develop caused either by the influenza virus or by bacteria infecting the damaged lung. Whatever the cause the presence of pneumonia is serious and the patient may die. Epidemics of influenza are common and may be severe. In the world-wide epidemic (pandemic) which occurred at the end of 1918 and beginning of 1919 more than 20 million people died. There are three types of influenza virus,

A, B and C, and type A strains are the principal cause of epidemics. Although patients develop protective antibodies the antigenic structure of the influenza virus may show major changes over years which render it insusceptible to attack by antibodies produced in response to an earlier infection. This change in the influenza virus also means that if influenza vaccines are to be effective they must be made from those strains of virus prevalent at the time and vaccination repeated as strains change.

Viruses which cause infections of the respiratory tract include the RESPIRATORY SYNCYTIAL VIRUS which is a cause of bronchitis and pneumonia particularly in children under one year of age, the PARA-INFLUENZA VIRUSES of which there are four types and which most commonly cause a cold with a high temperature and a cough, the ADENOVIRUSES of which there are 33 types and which can cause a sore throat, and the RHINOVIRUSES of which there are more than 100 and which cause common colds. Antibodies may be formed after an infection, but they are protective only against an attack by a virus of the same type.

MUMPS is an illness which usually occurs in childhood. The salivary glands are inflamed and swollen and other glands may also be affected such as the testes causing ORCHITIS and the pancreas causing PAN-CREATITIS. The disease is spread by inhalation of droplets of infectious saliva. As there is only one type of virus a person who has had an attack develops a good and long lasting immunity and second attacks rarely occur. A vaccine containing live attenuated virus is available.

MEASLES (p. 101) is the most common of the childhood fevers. It usually starts with an illness resembling a cold, but soon the characteristic rash appears. Although it is usually a mild disease complications, including a type of encephalitis, may be severe and vaccination with a vaccine containing live attenuated virus is recommended.

German measles, more properly known as RUBELLA, is normally a mild disease in which the patient who is usually under 15 years of age develops a temperature and a rash, but recovers completely within a few days. Many infections are symptomless. The importance of the disease lies in the fact that if it is contracted by a mother in the first 16 weeks of pregnancy the virus may cause congenital abnormalities in the foetus. Defects include cataracts, deafness, abnormalities of the heart and mental retardation. For this reason tests should be carried out on girls before they reach the child-bearing age or as soon as possible thereafter, to see if they have had rubella. Tests must be done as the patient will not know if she has had a subclinical infection and cannot be sure that an infection with symptoms was rubella. Blood is examined for antibodies to the virus. If they are present then the girl is immune and not liable to an attack in later life at a time when she might be pregnant. Patients who are not immune should be vaccinated with a live attenuated virus vaccine. Care must be taken not to vaccinate patients in early pregnancy.

HEPATITIS is inflammation of the liver and it may occur as a complication of several virus diseases. However, the most common types of hepatitis are known as Hepatitis A (infectious hepatitis) and Hepatitis B. The symptoms are similar in both conditions with jaundice, low grade fever and nausea. However, the two diseases are quite distinct.

In Hepatitis A the incubation period, that is the time between contact and the onset of the disease, is between two and six weeks. The virus is present in the faeces and the disease is transmitted when food, drink or other material containing the virus is swallowed. The onset is acute, but most people recover completely. Contacts of cases may be protected by giving them gamma–globulin (p. 46).

In Hepatitis B the incubation period is from two to five months. Although the virus may be present in a number of body secretions as well as the liver, in Britain the disease is usually transmitted by blood given as a consequence of a medical procedure such as blood transfusion. However, the amount of blood required to transmit the disease is minute, for example the quantity present on the tip of a needle or a hypodermic syringe if it is used on more than one patient without being sterilised between them. For this reason such a procedure must never be adopted and blood for transfusion is now tested for the presence of Hepatitis B surface antigen (HBsAg). This antigen, formerly known as Australia Antigen, is not the entire Hepatitis B virus, but probably part of it and an indicator of infectivity. Hepatisis B may be more severe than Hepatitis A and in some epidemics as many as 30% of those affected have died. The disease has caused particular problems and epidemics in renal transplantation and dialysis units. Following an infection patients may recover completely or become chronic carriers of the virus and therefore potentially infectious. Contacts cannot be protected with normal gamma–globulin, but gamma–globulin containing large amounts of antibody to HBsAg is of value and may be given to anyone who has a cut or scratch contaminated with blood from a patient suffering from the disease or a known HBsAg carrier.

CHLAMYDIAE

The chlamydiae are a group of closely related organisms which were previously considered to be viruses, but they are larger, being from 0.25 to 0.5μ in diameter, and may be stained and seen under the light microscope. Like viruses they can only multiply inside cells (OBLIGATE INTRACELLULAR PARASITES), but they have a complex life cycle which ends with binary fission. They contain both DNA and RNA and are sensitive to chloramphenicol, the tetracyclines and sulphonamide. Chlamydiae cause PSITTACOSIS (ornithosis), LYMPHOGRANULOMA VENEREUM, TRACHOMA and INCLUSION CONJUNCTIVITIS.

ORNITHOSIS is a disease of birds which is called PSITTACOSIS when it affects the psittacine ones (parrots and budgerigars). In birds it causes outbreaks of disease characterised by diarrhoea, emaciation and nasal discharge, but in man it causes atypical pneumonia (Chapter Twelve) when infected material from birds is inhaled. Naturally therefore the human disease is most common in people who keep birds as pets and pet shop owners.

LYMPHOGRANULOMA VENEREUM is a venereal disease seen only occasionally in Britain, but more common in the tropics. The main symptom is a swelling of the inguinal lymph glands (buboes) as a consequence of inflammation.

TRACHOMA and INCLUSION CONJUNCTIVITIS are both infections of the eye. TRACHOMA consists of inflammation of both the cornea and conjunctiva (kerato-conjunctivitis) and is often followed by scarring of the cornea. It is a major cause of blindness in tropical countries. INCLUSION CONJUNCTIVITIS is a milder form of conjunctivitis usually seen in neonates when it is acquired from the mother during birth, or in older people having been acquired by contact, for example in swimming pools. It generally resolves in three weeks. The agent may be found in the normal human genito-urinary tract in which it may cause no symptoms, but it may cause inflammation of the urethra (URETHRITIS) in males and inflammation of the cervix (CERVICITIS) in females.

Complement fixation tests can be done to assist in the diagnosis of all the chlamydial diseases and the agents can also be grown in special tissue cultures.

RICKETTSIAE

The RICKETTSIAE are a group of organisms which like the virus and chlamydiae are obligate intracellular parasites, but which contain both DNA and RNA and which have a structure more like that of Gram-negative bacteria. They are about 0.3μ in diameter, can be seen under the light microscope and are sensitive to chloramphenicol and tetracyclines. They can be studied by producing experimental infections in either laboratory animals, of which the guinea pig is commonly used, or by infecting living, fertile hens' eggs. In these ways they may be isolated from sufferers from the diseases which they cause. Such work is however attended with a considerable risk that the laboratory worker will himself become infected. Much more commonly the diagnosis of rickettsial infection is confirmed by the demonstration of the development of specific antibody in the patient's serum.

Rickettsiae cause a variety of human diseases including typhus, scrub typhus, rocky mountain spotted fever and Q fever. In most cases the rickettsial infection is transmitted to man by an insect. The insect either obtains the infection itself from a human case of the disease or from an animal carrying the disease. Thus epidemic typhus is spread by the bite of a louse, endemic typhus by the rat flea, scrub typhus by a particular type of mite. Q fever is in all probability not insect-spread, indeed the organism of this disease differs in other ways from the remainder of the RICKETTSIA and is often classified as a separate genus—COXIELLA. Q ('query') fever is a generalised infection with symptoms of headache and aches and pains. About half the affected patients develop atypical pneumonia (Chapter Twelve) and another complication is endocarditis.

As already mentioned the rickettsial diseases are usually diagnosed by the demonstration of the specific antibody response. This may be carried out as a complement fixation test against Rickettsia grown in the hen's egg, but a simpler, though not so satisfactory a method, is also available. It was found that certain strains of the Gram-negative bacillus *Proteus* were agglutinated by the serum of patients recovering from typhus. This is because they happen to contain antigens very similar to those possessed by the typhus-Rickettsia. Agglutination of three strains of *Proteus* by serum from patients with Rickettsial diseases is known as the WEIL-FELIX REACTION. It is not of value in all diseases caused by Rickettsiae, but is very useful in the diagnosis of typhus and scrub typhus.

Chapter Sixteen

ELEMENTARY PARASITOLOGY

Parasitology is the study of animals which live inside or on the surface of other animals, and which derive benefit from this habitat at the expense of the host animal. It is usual to exclude bacteria from a study of parasitology though they do in fact fit the definition. In this chapter we are only concerned with human parasites, although in the case of some parasites of man another animal host is involved in the life history. Parasites often have very complicated life histories, and may spend a part of their life in several different animals. The animal in which the parasite reaches the adult stage is known as the DEFINITIVE HOST, whilst hosts which sustain the earlier (larval) stages of parasite development are known as SECONDARY HOSTS. Parasites are sometimes divided into those which live on the surface of the host—ECTOPARASITES, and those which live inside the host body—ENDOPARASITES.

ECTOPARASITES OF MAN belong to the large group of jointed limbed animals, the *Arthropoda*. This group includes the crabs, lobsters, centipedes, spiders, insects, etc. Parasites of man within this group are the mites, ticks and insects. Ectoparasites are usually biting animals which require blood as a food. In some cases the blood feed is required only once in the life of the parasite, in others several or many feeds are usual.

The ectoparasites of man are important for several reasons. Firstly they may act as agents in the transmission of infection. Some of the infections which are transmitted by ectoparasites are shown in Table 2.

TABLE 2

DISEASES TRANSMITTED BY ECTOPARASITES

PARASITE	DISEASES
Flea	Plague, endemic typhus
Louse	Epidemic typhus
Tick	Many rickettsial infections
Mite	Scrub typhus
Mosquito	Malaria, yellow fever, encephalitis, other virus diseases
Biting flies	Sleeping sickness, kala-azar, sand fly fever.

Secondly ectoparasites may also cause harm to man by invading the skin. The itch mite which causes scabies is an example of this type of damage. In addition, the itching produced by frequent biting by mosquitos, flies, etc., in itself constitutes a considerable nuisance. Figure 16 illustrates the appearance of several important ectoparasites of man.

ENDOPARASITES may live in various situations in man. They may exist in the blood, in the tissues, in the lymph vessels and in the gastro-intestinal tract. Most human endoparasites are either single-celled animals—*Protozoa*, or various types of worms. The worms may be divided into FLAT WORMS (*Platyhelminthes*) and ROUND WORMS (*Nemathelminthes*). The flat worms include the flukes and the tape worms. We will first consider examples of parasitic protozoa and then discuss some of the more important parasitic worms.

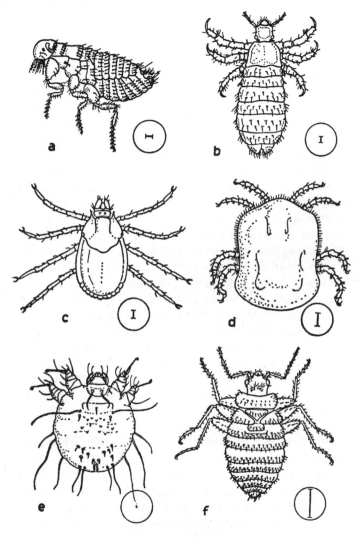

FIG. 16. Ectoparasites of man.

(a) Flea, (b) Louse, (c) Hard tick, (d) Soft tick, (e) Mite (scabies), (f) Bug. The small line enclosed in the circle next to each parasite indicates its approximate life size.

PARASITIC PROTOZOA

The examples of parasitic protozoa selected for discussion are *Plasmodium*, the causative agent of malaria which is a blood parasite. *Entamoeba histolytica*, a parasite of the intestine which causes amoebic dysentery, and *Trichomonas vaginalis* which causes infections of the female genital tract.

MALARIA is a disease which occurs in tropical and subtropical countries. The protozoa which cause malaria belong to the genus *Plasmodium*, and there are several species—*P. vivax, P. falciparum, P. ovale*, and *P. malariae*—which can be identified and which cause different types of the disease. Malaria is transmitted to man by the female ANOPHELES MOSQUITO. This genus includes many different species. The mosquito becomes infected by the *Plasmodium*, which undergoes part of its life history in the tissues of the mosquito. The rest of the life history is carried out in human tissues, notably in the red cells of the blood. The life cycle of *Plasmodium* then requires two hosts—man and the mosquito, in order that it may be complete. The link between the two hosts is the bite of the mosquito. If man is bitten by a mosquito infected with *Plasmodium* there is an incubation period of about two weeks before symptoms occur, during which the injected parasites live inside tissue cells in the liver. They leave the liver and enter the red cells of the blood where they develop from tiny objects (*trophozoites*) into much larger ones which almost fill the red cell (*schizonts*). The large form divides into many smaller forms (*merozoites*) which break out of the cell. This coincides with the clinical attack of malaria in which the patient's temperature rises, he alternately feels cold and shivers, and hot and sweats profusely. The merozoites released from the red cell infect other cells and the cycle continues again. It will be noted that reproduction of the *Plasmodium* is asexual during this cycle, and as the time taken to carry out this cycle is constant the attacks of malaria occur at regular intervals, each time related to the bursting out of the merozoites. The time for the cycle is 48 hours in *P. vivax* infections, 72 hours in *P. malariae* infections, and slightly less than 48 hours in *P. falciparum* infections. *P. vivax* infections are for this reason called TERTIAN MALARIA—attacks on the first and THIRD days; *P. malariae* infections with attacks on the first and FOURTH days are known as QUARTAN MALARIA, and *P. falciparum* infections with attacks at just less than 48 hour intervals are known as SUBTERTIAN MALARIA, or more commonly as MALIGNANT TERTIAN MALARIA because it tends to be more severe than *P. vivax* BENIGN TERTIAN malaria.

Some time after the asexual cycle has become established in man some of the parasites develop into male and female cells. These have no part to play in the human infection, but are necessary for the continuation of the life cycle in the mosquito. If the male and female cells are taken up by the mosquito in a blood meal, fertilisation of the female cells takes place and further development occurs in the mosquito tissues. The fertilised cell penetrates the stomach wall of the mosquito where it enlarges and multiplies to form a cyst containing numerous small structures—*sporozoites*. The sporozoites leave the cyst in the stomach wall and migrate to the mosquito's salivary glands. If the mosquito bites man at this stage the sporozoites are injected into the human tissues and the cycle is completed.

The diagnosis of malaria is confirmed by finding the parasite in stained films of blood. The species may also be determined by this means. Because the number of parasites may be small it is usual to examine a thick film of blood prepared by spreading several drops over an area of a microscope slide about 13 mm (½ in) in diameter. This is allowed to dry and then examined by a special method. Figure 17 shows the appearance of some stages of the malaria parasite whilst in the human red cell.

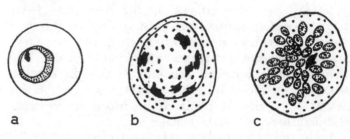

a   b   c

FIG. 17. Malaria parasites.

(a) Ring form within a red blood corpuscle (trophozoite), (b) A later stage within the red cell (schizont), (c) Division of the schizont to produce many merozoites which will now burst out of the cell.

Treatment of malaria is usually carried out with chloroquine, but chloroquine resistant organisms are common in some countries and then other drugs must be used. Control and prevention of malaria are important public health duties in malarious areas of the world. The chain of infection may be attacked at several points. Adult mosquitos are destroyed by the use of insecticides, and the larval stages of the mosquito are killed by treating the water in which they live with oil. In addition, wherever possible the mosquitos are denied the water they require for breeding by drainage schemes. Mosquitos are prevented from biting man by the use of fine mesh screens at doors and windows and by the use of mosquito netting over beds. The drug paludrine if taken daily will usually prevent the development of the malaria parasite in man even in an area in which malaria–infected mosquitos abound, although other drugs may sometimes be needed. By the use of such methods some areas of the world in which malaria was common are now completely free of the disease.

AMOEBIC DYSENTERY is an infection of the large intestine with the protozoal parasite *Entamoeba histolytica*. The disease is common in tropical and subtropical countries, but may be found almost anywhere in the world. The parasite does not require a secondary host, and infection is transmitted by food and water contaminated with the faeces of sufferers or carriers. Particularly important are salads, which in some countries are grown in soil fertilized with human faeces. Cooked foods are safe. The parasite lives in the mucous membrane of the large intestine in which it produces ulceration. The symptoms are chronic intermittent diarrhoea, often with some abdominal pain. Occasionally the parasite spreads from the large intestine to produce abscesses elsewhere in the body. The most common site is in the liver, but other sites are sometimes involved. Diagnosis of amoebic dysentery is confirmed by identifying the parasite in the faeces. This may prove difficult particularly in the very chronic case. The parasite may be present in the faeces as the active *vegetative form* or as a *cyst*. The appearance of these forms is illustrated diagrammatically in Fig. 18. The typical appearances of the vegetative forms of *E. histolytica* disappear when the temperature of the

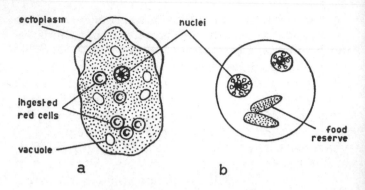

FIG. 18. *Entamoeba histolytica*.
(*a*) Vegetative stage, (*b*) Cyst stage.

faeces falls after passing. For this reason the specimen should be examined in the laboratory within minutes of being passed. As there are other species of amoeba which may be found in the faeces, and which appear to cause no harm, considerable skill is required in identifying *E. histolytica*. Metronidazole is used in the treatment of amoebic dysentery.

The third protozoan parasite to be considered is *Trichomonas vaginalis*. This produces an infection of the vagina which results in an offensive vaginal discharge. The disease is fairly common and in some cases, though not necessarily all, is transmitted by sexual contact. The same organism may be isolated from the urethra of the male, where it produces either no symptoms at all or a mild urethritis. Diagnosis of *T. vaginalis* infection is made by finding the typical parasite in the discharge. It is a large protozoan which moves by means of flagella. The parasite is illustrated in Fig. 19. Culture methods are available to detect the parasite when so few are present that visual detection is difficult. This method is of value in isolating the parasite from the male urethra. Treatment consists of metronidazole administered orally.

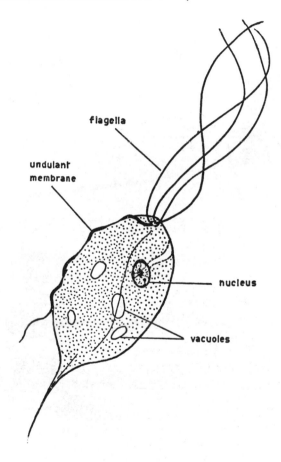

Fig. 19. *Trichomonas vaginalis.*

PARASITIC WORMS

There are very many different species of 'worm' which may parasitise man. They may be found in the gastro-intestinal tract, in the urinary tract, in the lymphatics, in the subcutaneous tissues and in the liver. Only four common species will be considered, all of which are found in this country. These are the tape worms *Taenia* and *Echinococcus*, the round worm *Ascaris* and the thread worm *Enterobius*.

Taenia is a genus of tape worms which has two

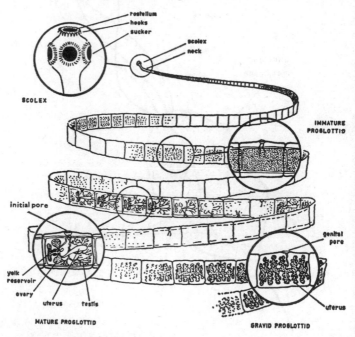

FIG. 20. The tape worm *Taenia solium*.

The inset figures show the detailed structure of the parasite.

species able to infect man. These are *T. solium* and *T. saginata*. They are very similar in appearance, but may be differentiated on detailed examination. The worms have a head, which in the case of *T. solium* has small hooks, and in both worms suckers, a neck, and below this a series of *proglottids* or segments (see Fig. 20). Each proglottid is a reproductive unit in itself. The proglottids are formed continuously at the neck of the worm and are pushed towards the rear end by the development of more new ones. The proglottids in the middle of the worm are larger and sexually mature. They contain both male and female sex apparatus. Fertilisation of the female cells takes place, and the proglottis becomes filled with fertilised ova. At the rear end of the worm the proglottids are largest, and consist almost entirely of a uterus filled with ova. The whole worm will consist of several hundred proglottids often resulting in a total length of several feet. The rearmost proglottids are shed in the faeces.

Both *T. saginata* and *T. solium* live in the human intestine where quite often they remain undetected. Symptoms which may be produced if the number of worms is large are anaemia and loss of weight. The mature proglottids and free ova are shed in the faeces, and the patient's complaint is more likely to be the finding of a proglottid, than actual illness. Diagnosis is confirmed by identifying a proglottid, or by finding ova of Taenia on microscopic examination of the faeces. The second stage of the life history takes place in either the pig (*T. solium*) or in cattle (*T. saginata*). If fertile ova are eaten by these animals, they hatch and larvae emerge which penetrate the wall of the intestine and migrate by way of the blood and the lymph to the muscles, where they encyst. The cysts remain in the muscle until the meat is eaten in an uncooked or partially cooked state when they develop into the adult worm and attach themselves by means of the hooks and/or suckers to the intestinal wall. The encysted stage of *T. solium*, which normally is found in pig muscle, may occasionally occur in man. This is brought about by the ingestion of fertile eggs by man. The stages of the life cycle which normally take place in the pig now occur in man. The disease is known as *cysticercosis*. Cysts may be found in many organs, but are most serious when present in the brain or the eye.

Treatment of tape worm infection is directed towards damaging the worm so that it may be passed in the faeces. Niclosamide or mepacrine, a drug originally used in the treatment of malaria, usually give satisfactory results. It is most important to ensure that the head is passed otherwise a cure cannot be guaranteed. All the faeces passed should be closely examined for the presence of the head by washing them through a fine mesh sieve.

Echinococcus granulosus is the dog tape worm and although the natural secondary host is the sheep, man may sometimes act as accidental secondary host. The ova are shed from the mature tape worm into the intestine of the dog and pass out with the faeces. If taken in by mouth either by man or the sheep, the fertilised ovum develops into a cystic stage known as a bladder worm. In man this is usually known as a *hydatid cyst* and occurs most commonly in the liver, but also sometimes in the lung. Dogs become infected by eating infected sheep tissues. The infection occurs particularly in sheep-farming communities where there is an intimate association of man, the dog, and sheep. Skin tests (Casoni test) and tests for antibodies are used to confirm the diagnosis of hydatid cyst. The drug mebendazole may shrink or kill hydatid cysts and avoid the need for their surgical removal.

Ascaris is a large round worm which usually measures approximately 15 cm (6 in) long by 0·6 cm (¼ in) in diameter. It is pointed at both ends, and is yellowish–grey in colour. Males and females may be recognised by detailed examination, the female being larger than the male. *Ascaris* infections are common throughout the world, particularly in children. Symptoms are not common, but may include anaemia. The commonest presentation is the passage of the adult worm in the faeces, or the vomiting of a worm. The adult worm lives in the small intestine, on occasions in large numbers. Mating takes place, and large numbers of ova are shed into the intestinal contents which are easily seen on microscopic examination of the faeces. There is no secondary host in the life history of *Ascaris*. The ova, if shed on to moist warm earth, pass through a stage of maturation which lasts about a month. The ova are now infective to man if eaten. Transference to man is brought about by soil contamination of vegetables, and in children by dirty fingers. After ingestion, a larva emerges from the ovum, passes through the intestinal wall, invades a blood vessel and so reaches the liver. It next migrates to the lungs, enters a bronchus and passes by way of the trachea into the oesophagus and thence into the intestine where it develops into the adult stage. During the passage of the larvae through the lungs there may be transient cough, sometimes with blood–stained sputum. There are several substances available for the treatment of *Ascaris* infections. A very satisfactory drug is piperazine which is taken by mouth.

Enterobius is a small round worm measuring less than 2·5 cm (1 in) in length. Its common name is the THREAD WORM or pin worm. Infection with this worm is very common especially in children. The worm is found attached to the mucosa of the intestine where mating takes place. The fertilised female worm now migrates to the rectum and anal canal and deposits the ova on the peri-anal skin. This causes intense itching, especially at night, which is the predominant symptom of thread worm infection. The ova when deposited contain a coiled larva, and unlike *Ascaris* require only a short time before they become infective. Commonly the ova are transferred to the person's fingers during scratching, and thence to the mouth. Thus there is a tendency for the infection to be perpetuated once established. There is no complex migration of the larva as in some other round worm life histories, and the *Enterobius* larva merely becomes adult on the way down the small intestine and attaches to the mucosa. It is unusual to find the ova in the faeces, but they may be seen in scrapings from the peri-anal skin. A useful method is to apply a strip of Sellotape to the peri-anal skin, sticky side innermost. When peeled off and examined microscopically the ova are usually easy to see.

If self re-infection can be stopped the worms die within a few months, and the infection is thus cured. It is unfortunately almost impossible to prevent a child from scratching, especially at night. Methods which are adopted include the use of gloves and one-piece night clothing. Piperazine is a valuable specific form of treatment, and it is usually essential to treat the whole family simultaneously, as adults often have symptomless infections.

GLOSSARY

Abscess
A localised collection of pus within the body tissues.

Acid-fast bacillus
An organism usually a member of the genus *Mycobacterium* which, when once stained, will resist decolorisation with acid.

Agglutination
The sticking together of particles (bacteria, etc.) by specific antibody which reacts with antigen present on the surface of the particles.

Alpha haemolysis
The green discoloration of the medium produced by some bacteria when grown on blood agar (*see* beta haemolysis).

Anaerobe
A micro-organism which will grow in the absence of oxygen.

Active immunity
Specific resistance to infection induced by previous contact with the infective agent or its products.

Antibiotic
A substance produced by a bacterium or a fungus which has a destructive activity against other micro-organisms.

Antibody
A type of protein, found in the blood, which will combine specifically with the antigen which induced its formation.

Antigen
A substance, most commonly either a protein or a polysaccharide, which will induce antibody formation in an animal if suitably presented (usually injected).

Anti-toxic immunity
Immunity to infection which

depends on the presence of circulating antibody (anti-toxin) which can neutralise the toxin of the infecting agent.

Anti-toxin   An antibody which can specifically neutralise a particular toxin.

Acquired immunity   Specific immunity to infection which may be acquired during life, either naturally or artificially (*see* innate immunity).

Arthropoda   The large group of animals characterised by having a hard outer skeleton (exoskeleton) and jointed limbs. The group includes crabs, lobsters, insects, spiders, etc., and is of interest to bacteriologists because some members of the group transmit human disease.

Attenuated strain   A strain of micro-organism which has diminished virulence as a result of various laboratory procedures.

Autoclave   A device in which objects are sterilised by steam under pressure.

Bacillus   A general term for a rod-shaped bacterium. Also the name of a genus of aerobic spore-bearing rod-shaped bacteria, e.g. *Bacillus anthracis*, the causative agent of anthrax.

Bacteraemia   The transient presence of bacteria in the blood.

Bacteriophage (*phage*)   A special type of virus which is able to infect and destroy bacteria. Phages are very host-specific and will often only attack certain strains of a particular bacterial species. Because of this phages are used to type bacteria.

Beta haemolysis	The complete clearing of the red cells in a blood–agar plate around a colony of certain bacteria, notably some types of *Streptococcus* (*see* alpha haemolysis).
Binary fission	Multiplication of micro–organisms by division to form two daughter cells.
Broth	Simple liquid medium used to grow bacteria in the laboratory.
Capsule	The outer mucoid layer of some bacteria. The capsule is outside the cell wall.
Carrier	A person who, though not suffering obviously from a particular disease, continues to harbour and to excrete the causative organisms which he may pass on to others.
Caseation	The soft cheesy material which is found in tissues destroyed by tuberculous inflammation.
Cellulitis	A diffuse inflammation of a tissue in which the inflammatory exudate does not usually localise to form pus, but which is spread evenly in the tissue spaces.
Cell mediated immunity	Resistance to infection achieved through the action of certain cells.
Cell wall	The firm outer layer of a bacterial cell which gives the organism its shape. (N.B. if the organism possesses a capsule this will be outside the cell wall.)
Chemotherapeutic agent	A synthetic substance which has a destructive action against micro-organisms, and which is used to treat infection.
Chlamydiae	Organisms similar to viruses, but

	which are slightly larger and contain two sorts of nucleic acid.
Coccus	A spherical bacterial cell.
Colony	A visible group of bacterial cells growing together on a solid bacteriological medium. They are usually assumed to have developed from a single cell by multiplication.
Conjugation	A para-sexual method of exchange of genetic material in bacteria.
Consolidation	The firmness found in the lung in pneumonia due to the air spaces being filled with inflammatory exudate.
Cystitis	Inflammation of the bladder.
Dark ground microscopy	A method of microscopy which allows unstained micro-organisms to be seen.
Dry heat sterilisation	A method of sterilisation by heating in an oven, usually to a temperature of 160°C for 1 hour.
Ectoparasite	A parasite which lives on the surface of its host, e.g. a flea.
Encephalitis	Inflammation of the brain tissue.
Encephalomyelitis	Inflammation of the brain and spinal cord.
Endoparasite	A parasite which lives inside its host, e.g. malaria parasite.
Erythrogenic toxin	A toxin produced by *Streptococcus pyogenes* which is responsible for the skin rash of scarlet fever.
Erysipelas	A spreading inflammation of the skin caused by *Streptococcus pyogenes*.
Facultative anaerobe	A micro-organism which can grow under both anaerobic and aerobic conditions.
Fermentation	The incomplete splitting of sugars by micro-organisms to provide

energy for their growth and which yields alcohols, acids and gases. Oxygen is not necessary for the reaction.

Flagellum   A whip-like structure which projects from the cell wall of certain bacteria. The bacterium is able to move by waving the flagella (plural).

FTA—ABS test   Absorbed fluorescent *Treponema pallidum* immobilisation test. A serological test used in the diagnosis of syphilis.

Gamma-globulin   The portion of serum proteins which contains the antibody activity. Human pooled gamma-globulin is used to produce passive immunity to some diseases.

Gas gangrene   An infection, usually of muscle, which is characterised by death of tissue and the production of a large amount of gas which distends the infected part. The causative organisms are members of the genus *Clostridium*.

Genus   A group of animals or plants (or bacteria) which, though not identical, have many characters in common.

Gram stain   A method of bacteriological staining which divides bacteria into Gram-positive and Gram-negative types. The Gram reaction depends on the nature of the bacterial cell wall.

Growth factor   A substance which needs to be present in small amounts in order to grow certain species of bacteria in

	artificial media. May be considered as bacterial vitamins.
Heaf test	A skin test for the detection of past or present tuberculous infection. A Heaf gun is used to inject tuberculin into the skin.
Hypersensitivity	A state in which a person or an animal responds in an unexpectedly vigorous and damaging way to a substance which would not be expected to cause such a reaction.
Innate immunity	The resistance to infection which is inborn in the animal and is not acquired either naturally or artificially.
Interferon	A substance released by cells infected with viruses which renders other cells resistant to virus infection.
Kahn test	A serological test used in the diagnosis of syphilis.
Lymphadenitis	Inflammation of a lymph node.
Lymphocyte	A small cell found in the blood and in lymphoid tissue (lymph nodes, the spleen, etc.); found also in chronic inflammation.
Macrophage	A large cell which has the ability to ingest (phagocytose) bacteria and other particles; found in chronic inflammation.
Mantoux test	A test for the detection of past or present tuberculous infection by the injection of tuberculin into the skin using a very fine needle and syringe (*see* Heaf test).
Medium	The mixture of substances in or on which bacteria are cultivated in the laboratory.

Meninges	The membranes which surround the brain and spinal cord.
Meningitis	Inflammation of the meninges.
Microaerophilic	Bacteria which grow best in the presence of a low concentration of oxygen, i.e. less than that found in air.
Micron	A unit of measurement of length; equals 1/1000th of a millimetre.
Moist heat sterilisation	Sterilisation in the presence of water, or steam. Boiling, steaming, and the use of pressurised steam in an autoclave are examples of this type of sterilisation.
Motile	Able to move under its own power.
Mutation	The spontaneous, random change which sometimes occurs in the genetic constitution of an organism. The change, having taken place, may be inherited by the progeny.
Mycoplasma	Organisms which structurally resemble bacteria except that they have no cell wall.
Myelitis	Inflammation of the spinal cord.
Native immunity	Resistance to infection which is not acquired during life, but is inherent in that species of animal.
Non-motile	Unable to move by its own power.
Normal flora	The micro-organisms which are found on the skin, in the respiratory tract, in the intestines etc., of the normal healthy animal (including man).
Otitis	Inflammation of the ear.
Parasite	An animal (or plant or micro-organism) which depends on some other living animal (or plant) to provide some or all the

	necessities for its life processes.
Passive immunity	Immunity which does not depend on the active participation of the animal so immune. The transfer of antibody from mother to foetus with the result that the newborn is immune to some diseases to which its mother is immune is an example of passive immunity.
Pathogenic	Disease-producing.
Peritonitis	Inflammation of the membrane lining the abdominal cavity and covering the viscera.
Petri dish	A shallow dish with a lid into which a solid bacteriological medium is placed for the cultivation of bacteria.
Phagocyte	A cell which can ingest particles including bacteria. Macrophages and polymorphonuclear leucocytes are examples of phagocytes.
Phagocytosis	The process of ingestion of particles by phagocytes.
Plasmids	Small fragments of deoxyribonucleic acid separate from the chromosomes of bacteria.
Pleurisy	Inflammation of the pleura (the membranes which line the thorax, and which cover the lungs).
Polymorph	Abbreviation in common use for polymorphonuclear leucocyte. A cell found in the blood which is a phagocyte and is very important as a first-line defence against bacterial invasion.
Primary chancre	The first stage of syphilis; a painless ulcer with thickened edges.
Primary complex	The tissue changes of the first stage

of tuberculous infection in a person who has never experienced the disease before. The complex includes the area of primary inflammation together with the inflamed lymph vessels and local lymph nodes.

Prophylaxis Prevention; usually used as in prophylaxis of disease—prevention of disease.

Protozoa Single-celled animals. Does not include bacteria and viruses which are nearer to the plant than the animal kingdom.

Purulent exudate The products of acute inflammation. The exudate is made up of blood proteins and inflammatory cells.

Pyaemia Literally—'pus in the blood'; the presence of aggregates of bacteria and inflammatory cells in the blood resulting in the presence of numerous secondary abscesses.

Pyelitis Inflammation of the pelvis of the kidney.

Pyelonephritis Inflammation of the pelvis of the kidney with spread to the kidney substance.

Pyogenic Literally—'pus producing'; usually applied to an infection in which pus is produced.

Respiration The process whereby complex chemical substances are broken down to simpler ones with the liberation of energy which may be used by the organism. The breakdown may or may not require the presence of oxygen.

Rickettsiae Organisms which are like small

bacteria which only multiply inside cells.

Saprophyte   A micro-organism which is able to live without parasitising an animal or a plant. It is not directly dependent on some other life form for the provision of the necessities of life.

Sensitivity test   A laboratory test to determine to which antibiotics an organism is sensitive, i.e. which antibiotics will either kill it or inhibit its growth.

Septicaemia   The result of failure of the body defences to contain a bacterial invasion with the result that bacteria multiply in the blood and their products (including toxins) are distributed about the body by the blood stream.

Species   A group of micro-organisms (or plants, or animals) which have very many characters in common; they are identical or near identical. There may be minor variations in some characters which are known as intra-species variation or strain differences.

Species immunity   Resistance to infection by a particular micro-organism which is an inherited character of a species of animal.

Spirillum   A spiral shaped organism with a rigid cell wall which is motile by means of flagella.

Spirochaete   Slender spiral organisms which are flexible, and which are motile without possessing flagella.

Spore   A structure produced by some species of bacteria which is very resistant to adverse conditions, e.g. heating or drying, which would kill the average bacterium. The spore is able to survive the adverse conditions and to germinate once conditions are favourable and so re-establish a bacterial population.

Stain
A dye used in bacteriology to colour micro-organisms and so make them more easily visible when examined microscopically.

Sterilisation
A process whereby all the living micro-organisms present on an object or in a liquid are destroyed or removed.

Sub-clinical infection
An infection with a pathogenic micro-organism which fails to produce the expected symptoms and so is not normally detected by the sufferer.

Synthesise
To make; to build up complex substances from simpler ones.

Toxaemia
The presence of toxins in the circulation, producing general symptoms and, in the case of some toxins, producing damage to certain target tissues.

Toxin
A substance produced by a micro-organism which has a damaging action on the tissues of a susceptible animal.

Toxoid
A toxin which has been treated to render it no longer toxic, but still able to induce anti-toxin formation if injected into an animal.

TPI test
Treponema pallidum immobilisation test. A serological test used in the diagnosis of syphilis.

Tissue culture   A system for growing virus.

Vaccine   A preparation of living or dead micro-organisms or of toxoids which when injected or in some other way presented to an animal or to man results in specific antibody formation and some measure of resistance to the appropriate infection.

VDRL test   Venereal Diseases Reference Laboratory Test. A serological test used in the diagnosis of syphilis.

Vibrio   A bacterium shaped as a curved rod, rather like a comma.

Virulence   An expression of the efficiency of a pathogenic micro-organism in causing disease. Virulence is very difficult to measure, but an estimate may be obtained by determining the minimum number of organisms which will cause the death of an animal into which they are injected.

Virus   A minute, microscopically invisible parasite containing only one sort of nucleic acid, DNA or RNA, and which can only multiply within the substance of the body cells of its host.

Wasserman reaction   A serological test used in the diagnosis of syphilis.

Weil-Felix reaction   A serological test used in the diagnosis of some Rickettsial diseases, notably in typhus and scrub typhus.

Widal test   A serological test used in the diagnosis of typhoid and paratyphoid.

Ziehl-Neelsen stain   A stain used to demonstrate acid-fast bacteria such as *Mycobacterium tuberculosis*.

INDEX

An asterisk after an entry in the index indicates that the word is included in the glossary.